Praise for

WHAT TO DO WHEN YOUR PARTNER IS DEPRESSED

"I love this book! Finally, here are practical, incredibly useful strategies for understanding your partner's depression and what you can do to help."

—John M. Gottman, PhD, coauthor of *Fight Right*

"Anyone who wants to improve their relationship with their loved one with depression should read this book! With clarity and compassion, Dr. Dozois shows how to provide emotional support while encouraging your partner to reengage with life."

—Judith S. Beck, PhD, President, Beck Institute for Cognitive Behavior Therapy

"When your partner is entangled with depressed mood and all it can bring, how can you stay connected without trying to 'fix' them? Dr. Dozois offers you a grounded, evidence-based way to respond—one that helps you promote meaningful change and care for yourself along the way. A compassionate and deeply practical guide."

—Steven C. Hayes, PhD, author of *Get Out of Your Mind and Into Your Life*

"You aren't your partner's therapist—but you can make a real difference in their recovery from depression. Dr. Dozois is a highly respected researcher and gifted clinician who brings years of wisdom to this excellent book. He gives you tools to be a better listener, communicator, and ally. The clear guidelines on setting limits and self-care are so essential for those supporting a partner."

—Robert L. Leahy, PhD, Department of Psychiatry, Weill Cornell Medical College; Director, American Institute for Cognitive Therapy

WHAT TO DO WHEN YOUR PARTNER IS DEPRESSED

Also Available

FOR PROFESSIONALS

Handbook of Cognitive-Behavioral Therapies, Fourth Edition
Keith S. Dobson and David J. A. Dozois, Editors

WHAT TO DO WHEN YOUR PARTNER IS DEPRESSED

Supporting Your Loved One While Caring for Yourself

DAVID J. A. DOZOIS, PhD

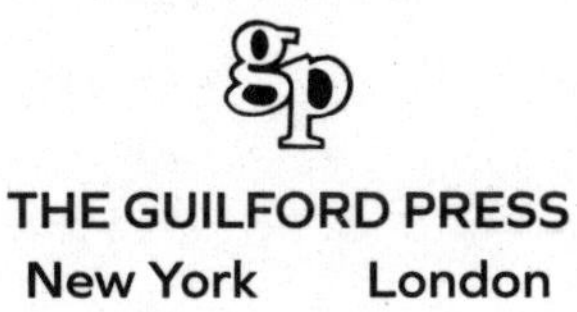

THE GUILFORD PRESS
New York London

A Division of Guilford Publications, Inc.
www.guilford.com

Printed in the United States of America

For product and safety concerns within the EU, please contact *GPSR@taylorandfrancis.com,* Taylor & Francis Verlag GmbH, Kaufingerstraße 24, 80331 München, Germany.

Last digit is print number: 9 8 7 6 5 4 3 2 1

Library of Congress Cataloging-in-Publication Data is available from the publisher.

ISBN 978-1-4625-5755-4 (paperback) — ISBN 978-1-4625-6361-6 (hardcover)

To my dad, John D. E. Dozois (1935–2025),
who, throughout his life, was a source of hope,
optimism, encouragement, and support

Contents

PART THREE
Supporting Your Relationship

PART FOUR
The Final Word

Acknowledgments

I would like to begin by thanking some of the collaborators, mentors, and colleagues who helped shape my thinking about vulnerability to depression and evidence-based psychological interventions and who impacted my research and practice over the years: Drs. Aaron Beck, Judy Beck, Deborah Dobson, Keith Dobson, Gene Flessati, Kate Harkness, Joelle LeMoult, Rod Martin, Kerry Mothersill, Andrea Piotrowski, Lena Quilty, Leslie Sokol, Lisa Starr, and Henny Westra.

I would also like to thank the team at The Guilford Press: Kitty Moore, who initially approached me about writing this book and whose vision made this book possible, and Christine Benton, who provided brilliant feedback and editing. It was wonderful to work with you both.

In addition, I would like to thank my parents, John and Judy Dozois, for their constant love, support, and encouragement; my sister, Elizabeth Dozois, whom I credit with initially teaching me how to write, many years ago when I was an undergraduate student; and the rest of my wonderful family who reside in Calgary, Alberta (Steve, Lindy, Caitlyn, Charlize, Elizabeth, Chris, Arden, Grady, Chayce, Christine, Theo, Hayden, August, and James); Winnipeg, Manitoba (Wanda, Richard, Ciocia, Steve, Kim, Luke, Katie); Toronto, Ontario (Mark, Christine, Landen, Adelaide); and southwestern Ontario (Rachel, Josh, Nora, Oakley, Asher, Joshua, and Kerstan).

I am especially grateful to my wife, Dr. Andrea Piotrowski, who has been an amazing source of encouragement, support, love, care, intellectual stimulation, fun, and laughter, and has helped me—to paraphrase Thoreau—suck the marrow out of life. Thanks also for providing feedback on my initial outline and an earlier draft of the book!

I would also like to thank the current members of the Breaking Sad Lab—my graduate students—Jennifer Gilles, Owen Hicks, Gabriela Murphy,

Sarina Rain, and Fei Ying. I would like to acknowledge some of the past members of my lab who have contributed importantly to my research, were a source of incredible encouragement, and made supervision such a rewarding experience: Roger Covin, Lindsay Evraire, Daniel Machado, Allison Ouimet, Katerina Rnic, Lindsay Szota, and Jesse Lee Wilde.

I am extremely grateful to the patients I have worked with over the years and from whom I have learned a tremendous amount. Thank you for trusting me. I have been deeply moved by your experiences and inspired by your resilience and courage.

Finally, I would like to thank the individuals who agreed to be interviewed for this book and who generously shared their stories with me.

Introduction

MAKING THE MOST OF THIS BOOK

Depression is brutal. It feels as though you've fallen into a dark, bottomless pit that seems impossible to climb out of. Every day the void gets bigger and bigger and the emptiness and hollowness become all consuming. And that's just the experience of the person with depression. When your partner is suffering with depression, you too feel the brunt.

Cynthia and her partner, Carlos, had been together for 10 years when she experienced her first episode of depression, following the onset of back pain that she started envisioning as permanent. As she described it, "The pain fed the depression, and the depression exacerbated the pain." Now Cynthia only feels numb, empty, sad, anxious, and hopeless. Nothing seems to make her happy, and she is distressed that she isn't presently capable of being the partner she had been, or intended to be, for Carlos. Carlos doesn't know what to do to help and keeps asking her when it's going to get better. Cynthia feels guilty that she is so frustrating and exhausting to live with, and Carlos feels guilty that he can't find a way to help. What can they do?

As a partner of someone with depression (or who you suspect may be depressed), you are likely experiencing a wide range of complex, conflicting, and confusing thoughts and emotions yourself: uncertainty, anxiety, sadness, helplessness, hopelessness, frustration, and disappointment. You may even be aware of some thoughts and feelings you don't care to admit to, like anger or resentment, or thoughts like "Hey, wait a minute. I didn't sign up for this!"

Being in a relationship with someone who is depressed can, itself, seem like a dark, endless path. Sabrina and her partner, Rick, have been together for 15 years and married for eight. Rick opened up about his depression at the start of their relationship, so Sabrina knew what she was getting into, or so she thought. But she didn't fully understand what this meant, how this would play out, or what impact depression would have on their relationship. They experienced lots of good times, but their relationship has also been rocky, layered with many obstacles and heartaches. Sabrina and Rick are currently seeing a couple therapist to sort out whether to stay together or separate and how best to move forward either way. Sabrina is also seeing a psychologist to process her own emotions and experiences. It has been a rough journey. What to do with all these difficult feelings?

These are only two stories out of millions and millions worldwide, and, like all the stories in this book, these are composites or fully disguised to protect privacy. They are meant to illustrate some of the pain, agony, and suffering that arise when you have a partner who is depressed. But, of course, the story of every couple is unique, including yours.

You may feel like your partner is in a deep, deep pit and you are looking down, trying to figure out how to get them out. From your perspective, they may be doing the best they can to claw their way out. Or maybe you don't think they have tried everything and are giving up, just sitting in the darkness, immobilized and hopeless.

What do you do? You may feel helpless. Do you call down and encourage your partner? Do you explain how *you* would climb out of the hole? Do you run and get help? You know that jumping into the pit will only make both of you stuck, and so you try to manage from above. You probably feel powerless. *If only my partner could improve. If only I could help get them out of the deep pit so we could get our lives back. If only things could go back to the way they were. If only. If only.* You recognize that what you really need are the proper tools—a long rope, a rescue pulley, perhaps a ladder—that will help them climb out of depression and allow you and your relationship to get back on track.

You likely picked up this book because you've tried in so many ways to help your partner, and you're feeling stuck. Or maybe you're not sure your partner is experiencing depression. Is your partner sad, fatigued, or hopeless much of the time? No longer interested in anything that once brought joy? Often feeling irritated, worthless, or ashamed? Whether or not your partner has been diagnosed, this book will show you what depression looks like, how it can be treated effectively, and what you can do to help both your partner and yourself. You may have just started this journey or been on the long and winding road for what seems like an eternity. Either way, you might be confused and paralyzed; you might be exhausted by figuring out how to take care of all the responsibilities your partner no longer handles, and neglecting your own health and care. In the following chapters I help you balance your partner's needs with your own and offer strategies for preserving your relationship without giving up on yourself.

TRY THIS: TAKE AN INVENTORY OF YOUR OWN QUESTIONS

Take a few moments to consider your own experiences. What is *your* story? What are you going through? Grab a pen and paper or device and jot down some of these experiences. A flood of questions is probably flying through your mind at this moment. Spend 5 or 10 minutes thinking about what questions you have. Elaborate on what some of these questions might be. This might help you make some sense of your experiences and know what to look for specifically in this book.

The questions that come up for most people I've known who have done this exercise are about their partner, themselves, or their relationship.

What came up for you about your partner?

- ❑ "Why is my partner acting like this? What is wrong with them?"
- ❑ "What happened to the person I first got together with?"
- ❑ "Why can't they get over this? How long will this last? Why can't I just get my partner back?"

You may be curious about what you can do to best support them:

- ❑ "My partner is so down all the time. What can I do to help lift their mood?"
- ❑ "How am I supposed to react to my partner's depression?"
- ❑ "How do I know if I am pushing too much or not enough?"
- ❑ "What strategies are most effective?"

What came up for you about yourself?

- ❑ "This isn't fair. I don't feel like I have a life. What can I do to help *me* through this process?"
- ❑ "Is it my fault?"

- ❑ "Am I being selfish for wanting to attend to my own needs?"
- ❑ "How do I put one foot in front of the other? How do I cope and get through this unscathed?"

And what about your relationship?

- ❑ "I don't feel like we connect anymore. What can I do to change that?"
- ❑ "How can we get our relationship back the way it was?"
- ❑ "Are there ways we can communicate better?"
- ❑ "How can our relationship grow and flourish despite my partner being enveloped in this darkness?"
- ❑ "What are we capable of changing? What can't we change and need to learn to accept?"
- ❑ "I know I said, 'for better or worse, in sickness and in health, till death do us part,' but is this worth all the heartache and pain?"

About This Book

This book is intended to answer questions like these, offering effective, evidence-based tools to support your partner, improve your own well-being, and enhance your relationship. The core message throughout is that by changing thoughts and behaviors you can optimally assist your partner, support yourself, and improve your relationship. There are no quick fixes—no gimmicks or simple solutions—but using the strategies in this book can help improve your partner's mood, which, in turn, will enhance your well-being and relationship satisfaction. You will also learn ways to cope and live as fully as possible, despite their depression, and engage in behaviors that optimize your relationship. I can't guarantee that this will be easy, but I will provide tips to support your efforts and help you honor your own needs as well as your partner's.

Avoidance can feel so much easier, but you probably have a clear sense that you need to deal with your partner's depression. Even if your partner improves, depression is unfortunately a highly recurrent disorder. If someone has a single episode of depression, the odds are about 50% that they will have a subsequent episode. After two episodes, the chance of having an additional episode is about 70%. It is closer to 90% for those who have had three or more episodes. So dealing with it now is important. This book can help your loved one get better and, equally important, have a better chance of staying well.

Everything in this book is based on scientific research and backed by numerous research papers, as well as my clinical work. I am a professor of psychology at Western University in London, Ontario, Canada, and a practicing doctoral-level psychologist. Both my research and my clinical expertise are focused on depression. This combination of science and practice, and my focus on depression, means that I am in a good position to let you know not only what the research evidence says works but how you can apply it practically to your everyday life.

I have seen the strategies in this book help hundreds of clients and show high rates of effectiveness in mountains of research. However, you should know that research on cultural diversity, same-sex couples, and gender diversity, although growing, is still sorely lacking. Therefore, although most of the strategies in this book should still apply and be helpful to you, if you find that any of them don't quite fit for you, you should feel free to adapt them (on your own or with the help of a therapist) so that they do work for you.

Part One is about learning how to optimally support your partner with depression. The chapters in this section can help you:

- Understand the experience of depression, including the thoughts, behaviors, and emotions that often accompany this problem
- Appreciate some of the common responses you may be experiencing and recognize that you are neither a bad person (or partner) for feeling them nor alone in them
- Provide support in ways that help you better communicate and connect with your partner
- Become informed about effective treatments
- Learn how to discuss your concerns and encourage treatment
- Work with your partner to engage in antidepressant behavior and reduce avoidance
- Help your partner change negative thinking
- Recognize warning signs and prepare for setbacks

As you no doubt have already experienced, depression is extremely difficult to contend with and puts an enormous strain on you and your relationship. Part Two will help you understand and process how you are feeling so that you can cope effectively and not continually drain the tank. The chapters in this section will help you:

- Make sense of your feelings and not lose yourself in the process
- Keep your own thinking in check to ensure that your mindset is as healthy as possible
- Understand that taking care of your own needs is not selfish
- Surround yourself with support and resources
- Put structure and routine back into your life

When we enter a romantic relationship, we expect that our partners will be there to provide support and stimulation, but sometimes they aren't able to make us feel loved and cared for or fail to show up. This is heart-wrenching. In Part Three I guide you through a set of strategies for managing relationship difficulties, improving your functioning as a couple, and ensuring that your relationship thrives even amid depression. The chapters in this section will help you:

- Understand how depression and relationship distress often go hand in hand
- Deal with thorny issues like navigating roles and responsibilities, managing feelings of rejection, or coping when it feels like love and sexual intimacy are on the rocks
- Learn to catch and change negative thoughts about the situation and your partner so you can improve intimacy and relationship quality
- Communicate and problem-solve more effectively as a couple
- Accept those things you can't change in your partner or in your relationship

Finally, Part Four emphasizes what to do when your partner's depression either has or hasn't improved. You will learn about relapse prevention, couple therapy options, and forgiveness. You will also read about finding meaning through suffering and maintaining hope.

Making the Best Use of This Book

To get back to the subject of this Introduction, here are a few tips for getting the most out of reading and using the ideas in this book:

- Check your commitment—to your partner and to investing the time and energy to support your partner and help them improve. I'm not advocating for blind self-sacrifice or exhausting yourself to the point of burnout. But if the love you've felt for your partner is alive and you want your relationship to survive, and the two of you to thrive within it, the strategies in this book are worth a shot. They won't all work for everyone, but some will become more effective with practice, and others can be replaced by alternatives given in this book. And if you're experiencing serious relationship distress, you might consider seeing a mental health professional for individual or couple therapy to work through these issues.

- Tell your partner that you are reading this book and will be trying out some new strategies in the service of supporting them, helping you cope, and bolstering your relationship. Sharing this information may help your partner feel understood and valued. It may also instill a sense of hope. If your partner expresses interest in reading it too, great, but don't exert any pressure on them to do so.

- Approach this book with an open mind. If you look at a strategy and immediately think *This will never work* because you've tried it before with no success or it sounds too simple, step back and see if you can find a time when you're willing to try it. If you give it a shot, chances are something will stick or you'll get a little bit of insight that can help you in another way. Mix things up a bit to freshen your perspective as well: try something again that didn't work a while back or experiment with something that you decided not to try, approaching the strategy from a different angle.

- Before moving on to the body of the book, please know that you will benefit most by starting at the beginning and reading through, pausing at different points to reflect on your experiences and working through different plans and recommendations. If you have a burning desire to jump to a particular section of the book you think might be more relevant and fruitful for you, go for it. I would just encourage you to come back and not skip other chapters, as they are each written to help you target different components of your partner's depression, your own well-being, and your relationship.

- Throughout your journey, above all, remember to be kind to yourself. This is not an easy road to travel, although it is usually a worthwhile trip. Give yourself permission to take care of yourself, meet your own needs, and get the support you deserve.

PART ONE

Supporting Your Partner

1

Understanding the Experience of Depression

What happened to my partner? How did they shift from being emotionally and physically available to being shut off? How is it that we used to communicate so well, but now they're retreating more and more? Why is talking about *anything* a massive chore? What happened to all the wonderful qualities that first attracted me to my partner?

You're likely very confused at this point, questioning not only what you can do to help but how long this will last, how you will manage, and whether your relationship will ever return to normal. Perhaps you're feeling demoralized or resentful about how your partner's depression is impacting you. Maybe you're blaming yourself for your partner's depression, wracking your brain about what you could have done differently to prevent this from occurring in the first place. These feelings are all perfectly reasonable. We will get to strategies soon. I promise. For now, let's begin to fit the pieces of the depression puzzle together.

Have you ever worked on a jigsaw puzzle? If so, you know there's a bit of strategy to it. First you need to flip the pieces up so you can see them. Then many people put the border of the puzzle together. Next they sort the pieces by color and shape and start working on small sections, which they then fit within the overall framework. Sometimes it's helpful to back up and see the bigger picture; at others it might help to take a break. The key is to keep chipping away and not give up.

Depression is kind of like a puzzle to solve. I get it—you don't want to view this is as your new hobby, but stick with me here. Much like the strategy for completing a puzzle, you need to start by seeing what's in front of you, flipping over the pieces to see what you're dealing with. Then you can work on some basic strategies that will help to support your partner, you, and your relationship. In this book, instead of worrying about how all of this is going to fit together, we'll focus on one small section at a time. Baby steps. Eventually your understanding will grow, and you'll have a set of new skills and strategies that you can put together and fit into the bigger picture.

At times you'll need to back up and get a different perspective. Sometimes a strategy you try isn't going to work and you might see it as a massive fail. That's no doubt upsetting but not catastrophic. Try to view failure as feedback, as part of the process. When something doesn't work out, it probably means you need to view the situation from a different angle to see how the pieces fit into the bigger picture of your partner's depression, your life, and your relationship. At other times you may need to cut your losses and try something completely different. Don't give up. You can do this. Your new puzzle strategy and persistence will pay off.

In this chapter, we start putting the pieces of the puzzle together by looking at the nature of depression and how this may show up in your partner's life. In other sections of the book we will focus on how to help yourself and your relationship.

Understanding what your partner is going through is critical for providing effective support. It allows you to see what's on the table. Knowing what you're dealing with and what to look for can better equip you to help your loved one. Moreover, gaining a grasp of these symptoms may help you better understand and accept some of the things that may be frustrating you about your partner and leaving you bewildered.

Let's say you walk into your home from work and start telling your partner about your day. Partway through what seems like a one-sided conversation you start to realize your partner has not really heard a word you've said. You might interpret this as lack of interest or lack of care from your partner. Or you might recognize that your partner's passive, muted response reflects their inability to concentrate—a symptom of depression.

Or maybe you've prepared a romantic evening together, complete with a special dinner, candles, and music, hoping to hint at your desire for closeness and sexual intimacy. But these attempts backfired and were only met with what felt like a cold shoulder. Understanding that lack of sex drive is related to symptoms of low energy and loss of interest, although still disappointing and frustrating, may help take the edge off or at least prevent you from taking it personally. By understanding the cluster of symptoms we call "depression," and recognizing their severity, you might even be able to see it from a different vantage point; one that views depression as an "it"—as a problem to be solved together with your partner, rather than something your loved one is doing intentionally to hurt you or a red flag that your relationship is falling through the cracks.

The objective is not to diagnose your partner or pin down precisely what they are experiencing but to gain a better understanding so that some of these experiences make some sense to you and feel a little less alien. By getting to know the beast that is depression, you might feel less resentment when your partner seems lethargic and isn't helping with household chores, refuses to join you at a social gathering, forgets something you said in a conversation, or retreats to the bedroom for frequent naps or time alone.

The Nature of Depression

We all have times when we feel like the air in our balloon is slowly deflating. On some days we just don't want to get out of bed or feel like facing the day. The losses, frustrations, failures, and disappointments of life can make everyone feel down or blue sometimes. For many of us, however, these feelings go away once we talk things through, do things we enjoy, or solve a particular problem. Because feeling morose is an experience we can all relate to, we tend to throw around the phrase "I'm feeling depressed" which, unfortunately, undermines what people with clinical depression are going through and contributes to misunderstanding what depression is truly about.

Clinical depression is more than just low mood. It is a mental disorder that involves overwhelming and enveloping despair. Depression is associated with significant impairments in how we think, feel, and behave and is intertwined with a host of physical symptoms that impair functioning.

Tina is 45 and has a 15-year history of depression. Her most recent episode of depression began a year ago, after she experienced increased stress at work. She worked for an accounting firm and had recently completed her educational requirements to become a chartered accountant when depression hit her like a Mack truck. She couldn't concentrate on her work and kept falling behind on assignments. Although her boss was understanding at first, frustration mounted when she kept missing deadlines. Tina felt like her brain was paralyzed. Her partner also noticed that Tina appeared to freeze and tense up when making even basic decisions like what to have for dinner or which TV show to watch. It got to the point where Tina wasn't able to maintain her attention on more than a couple of sentences of a magazine or newspaper and was quite unresponsive in conversation. She just seemed locked in the recesses of her mind, stewing repeatedly about her failures and beating herself up mentally, calling herself "stupid" and "incompetent." Tina was often tearful and felt utterly worthless and unlovable. Although her partner tried to reassure Tina that she was well loved, this information wouldn't sink in. Instead, it would seem to fly in one ear and out the other.

Because she felt little energy or motivation, Tina started avoiding things that previously gave her a sense of pleasure or a feeling of accomplishment. She no longer went for walks, read books, or gardened, which she used to enjoy immensely. Tina would often retreat to her room or space out in front of the television. She hardly ate. She had no appetite and was losing weight. At night she would lie in bed with her eyes wide open, tossing and turning for hours and hours. She had no interest in sex. In fact, her interest for most things was muted. Tina was constantly tired and felt as though every step was a major chore. She found it increasingly difficult to do even basic tasks like folding the laundry or washing the dishes. Although she was not actively suicidal, Tina did have thoughts like "You'd be better off without me" or "I wish I was never born."

When someone is depressed, several changes take place that affect their thinking, behavior, emotions, and physical well-being.

Negative Thinking

As for Tina, negative thinking is a common feature of depression. People who suffer from depression often beat themselves up for what they said or didn't say; what they did or didn't do. Although they aren't trying to be pessimistic, everything is viewed through a negative lens—how they see themselves, their perception of others, including you, and their outlook on their future. It's all so bleak, meaningless, discouraging, and hopeless.

When good things happen, your partner might chalk it up to luck, thinking that it is only short-lived and certainly not indicative of who they are or what they've accomplished. Conversely, when negative things occur, it's the total opposite. They see negative events as due to an inherent flaw in them, part of who they are. They think that bad things will only continue to occur in the foreseeable future. And it is not just this one thing that goes wrong; everything seems hopeless and negative. Perhaps you've noticed your partner is overly self-focused and constantly replaying negative things in their mind. They might be highly self-critical or overly harsh with themself or you.

Difficulty Thinking

You might also notice your partner's ability to think is impaired when they're in the grip of depression. They may have difficulty concentrating, remembering or following instructions, or completing tasks. They may be confused. Your partner may experience memory loss or have difficulty thinking of solutions to different problems. Because they aren't thinking as clearly as they normally would, they have difficulty making decisions or appear indecisive.

Changes in Behavior

You might also be aware of changes in how your partner acts, perhaps withdrawing from you, blocking out conversations, or avoiding being active. Maybe they seem to have a short fuse. You might see that they aren't really doing much of anything rewarding or enjoyable. Wanting to do less when feeling this way makes sense; they don't have the motivation or energy and feel constantly fatigued. Resting is wise when we've caught the flu, but with depression it becomes a double-edged sword. Retreating and hiding from the world only contributes to the very problem your partner is trying to avoid. It becomes a vicious, downward spiral.

Other behavioral signs include how your partner is moving and their mannerisms. Are they slower in walking or speech or, conversely, pacing and wringing their fingers and appearing agitated? Both can be signs of depression. Are they making less eye contact or acting less animated than usual? Research shows that individuals with depression make less eye contact, demonstrate slower speech, show more slumped posture, and exhibit fewer hand, head, and body movements during a conversation than people without depression. They may also engage less socially and may not show signs that they are interested in conversation, like smiling, raising their eyebrows, nodding, or laughing.

Shifts in Emotion

You may also notice a change in your partner's emotions. They might report feeling sad, empty, hopeless, or numb. Perhaps you've noticed they are despondent or that their eyes well up with tears on a regular basis. They may be restless, irritable, or anxious.

Physical Changes

Your partner might also be showing physical signs of depression like low energy and feeling tired all the time or exhibiting changes in their sleep patterns or appetite.

What Does It All Mean?

This may seem like a perplexing picture and one that is difficult to understand. To make matters worse, no objective test is available to diagnose depression as there is for pancreatitis or COVID. Psychologists certainly have important tools like structured diagnostic interviews and questionnaires that help determine whether someone meets diagnostic criteria for depression and to get a read on how severe their symptoms might be. But it's not as though you can draw blood and determine that your partner has depression or view them under a microscope and see, "Oh, there's the problem."

Instead, researchers and clinicians have studied which symptoms tend to go together consistently and reliably to make up this construct we call depression. A diagnosis of depression is made based on an assessment of all the symptoms your partner is experiencing and an understanding of how much these symptoms interfere with their life: work, relationships, level of distress, and so on. The criteria that mental health professionals use to diagnose depression are based on one of two standards: the *Diagnostic and Statistical Manual of Mental Disorders,* or DSM, published by the American Psychiatric Association and more commonly used in North America, or the *International Classification of Diseases* (ICD), published by the World Health Organization.

Understanding the various ways depression may show up can help you know what to keep an eye out for and grasp how debilitating this disorder can be. Getting a clearer sense of depression might also help you interpret your partner's thoughts, feelings, and behaviors in a different light, one that is empathic. Finally, appreciating what depression is and how it impacts your partner's life, you, and your relationship is an important first step toward making it better, which is the focus of subsequent chapters.

Types of Depression

Several different mental disorders have depression as a core feature and share common features such as sadness, loss of interest, emptiness, irritability, various physical symptoms, and negative thinking. The strategies described in this book will be helpful regardless of the specific ways depression shows up, but here are the diagnoses your partner might receive. If your partner hasn't been diagnosed, the following information may help you know when it's important for them to get a proper psychological assessment and treatment.

Major Depressive Disorder

Major depressive disorder (or what is commonly referred to as "clinical depression") is perhaps the most well-known. This disorder is characterized by sadness or markedly diminished interest or pleasure in most activities. Additional symptoms include feeling worthless or experiencing guilt that is extreme or out of proportion to the circumstances. Many individuals with depression also describe feeling numb or empty. People with major depression may also express thoughts of ending their lives or may make attempts to do so.

Some symptoms of depression are characterized by behaviors that are too little on one hand or too much on the other. For example, you may be noticing your partner moving or talking more slowly than is normal for them or revved up, anxious, and agitated, pacing back and forth as though they can't settle down. Individuals with depression also often experience problems with too little or too much sleep. Your partner may have also lost or gained weight or experienced a decrease or increase in appetite.

People with depression also frequently have difficulty concentrating, thinking clearly, or making decisions. Your partner may come across to you as indecisive or wishy-washy, for instance. They may regularly lose their train of thought and find it difficult to carry on a conversation. Or perhaps their attention is so impaired that they can't read a paragraph on their phone or e-reader.

Another common complaint involves loss of energy or fatigue. No matter what they do, your partner may constantly be feeling depleted and exhausted.

Psychologists or psychiatrists look for one of two cardinal symptoms—sadness or loss of interest—to diagnose major depression. It's important to understand that your partner may not express feelings of sadness but could still be clinically depressed. If your partner is expressing a significant and pervasive loss of interest or inability to experience pleasure in work, hobbies, activities or time with family and friends, depression may be the culprit.

So, if either of these symptoms plus any four of the others described are present nearly every day for a period of at least two weeks and cause notable distress or impairment, it might be major depression and would be worth exploring the option of getting professional help.

There are other variants of major depression as well. Many people, especially far from the equator, feel more sluggish and down when winter arrives. When clinical depression comes on particularly strong during the winter months, it is called seasonal affective disorder, or SAD.

Major depression can also occur around and following childbirth, a phenomenon called mood disorder with peri- or postpartum onset. Although having a child is usually associated with positive (albeit stressful) changes in one's life, as many as 70% of women experience mood swings and depression following pregnancy and childbirth. In most cases, the postpartum blues get better on their own and do not interfere with day-to-day functioning. In other instances, negative mood becomes chronic and severe enough that it results in a depressive episode (in rare instances, about 0.1% of the time, it can include psychotic symptoms if not treated effectively).

Persistent Depressive Disorder

With persistent depressive disorder, a person experiences sad mood for most of the day (more days than not) for a period of two years or longer. In addition to chronic sadness, this disorder presents other symptoms, including sleep problems, appetite changes, low energy, low self-esteem, poor concentration or trouble making decisions, and hopelessness. Many individuals with this problem can still function at work or school and may see their negativity simply as part of their gloomy personality. They might claim, "I have felt this way for as long as I can remember. It's just the way I am." These symptoms can last for years and impact relationships and other daily activities. Although persistent depressive disorder is typically less severe than major depression, it is not uncommon for people to slip into periods of more severe depression. In some cases, the persistence of a severe episode can also last for many years.

Depression Associated with Bipolar Mood Disorders

Bipolar disorders are characterized by periods of mania or hypomania. What is called bipolar I disorder (or used to be referred to as manic depression), involves a roller coaster of extreme highs of mania and extreme lows of depression. Mania occurs when there is a distinct period of feeling on top of the world, unstoppable, and invincible. Individuals who are in a manic state often experience inflated self-esteem, seem to have limitless energy, experience less need for sleep, and are much more talkative than usual, as though they are jumping from thought to thought to thought in rapid succession. When people are in a manic state, they may engage in reckless behaviors they wouldn't otherwise do like going on buying sprees or having sexual affairs.

One day my client Tom, who had bipolar disorder, stepped out onto his balcony and looked down 15 floors to the greenspace surrounding his apartment building. He could see that the lawn care providers were mowing the lawn; but they weren't doing it fast enough for his liking. So, he bought his own lawn mower. The lawn mower he bought wasn't doing a quick enough job, so he bought another lawn mower and then a third and a fourth. After his manic phase was over, Tom fell into a depression. He also felt embarrassed and overwhelmed by his reckless behavior. Living in a small apartment, he didn't need a single lawn mower let alone four of them!

Years ago I worked at a high-end jewelry store before going to university. I recall someone coming in and buying more and more items from the store; one after another after another. Rings, crystal vases, watches, necklaces. When the total amount purchased climbed past $20,000, the credit card company swiftly phoned the store and told us to confiscate and destroy the credit card.

Sometimes individuals in a manic episode can be extremely irritable or aggressive. This mood state lasts at least one week and is combined with other symptoms. Although some people experience only manic episodes and do not fall into the pit of depression, most individuals with bipolar I disorder oscillate between these extreme highs and the devastating lows of depression. Hospitalization is often necessary to help stabilize their mood state.

Bipolar II disorder involves at least one episode of major depression and at least one hypomanic episode, without a history of mania. Hypomania involves the same number of symptoms as mania but is less extreme than a full-blown manic episode, does not cause significant impairment, and lasts a minimum of four days.

Many individuals describe a manic or hypomanic state as enjoyable and productive. They have a ton of energy and can get a lot done. They often feel as though they are thinking more clearly and bursting at the seams with positive emotions. The downside is that this can lead them to ignore the serious consequences of their symptoms for their own lives or how their behaviors are negatively impacting others.

An individual with bipolar I disorder may seek treatment (or be brought in for treatment by police or their loved ones) when they are at either end of the spectrum of mania or depression, whereas individuals with bipolar II disorder usually seek treatment when they have hit rock bottom and are experiencing depression.

A related disorder, cyclothymia, involves a chronic but less severe form of bipolar disorder. Technically, there are at least two years of cycling between hypomania and depression that is less severe than a full major depressive episode.

Other Problems Related to Depression

Depression is frequently associated with other mental health problems and physical conditions. For example, about 60% of people with depression have a co-occurring anxiety problem like panic disorder, social anxiety, chronic worry, or trauma-related anxiety. There are also higher rates of substance use. Depression is also more likely when someone is experiencing medical conditions like chronic pain, cancer, cardiovascular issues, or hypothyroidism. To rule out physical causes or conditions that might mimic depression, it is important to get a thorough assessment. A medical and psychological assessment will also help your partner figure out the optimal treatment plans. For example, would it make sense to deal with the anxiety first and then depression or the other way around?

TRY THIS: CONSIDER YOUR PARTNER'S SYMPTOMS

What symptoms of depression have you noticed in your partner? How has this impacted them? How has it impacted you? Take a moment to reflect on these symptoms. See if you can determine what might be due to depression (rather than who they are or a signal that the relationship is hitting rock bottom). Does this help to personalize it less and increase your compassion and empathy for your partner?

Why Is My Partner Depressed?

When depression strikes a couple, both of you can feel very alone, very frustrated by the disorder's impact.

"Why Me? Why Us?"

The truth is you and your partner are not alone. Depression is so ubiquitous that it is often termed the "common cold" of mental disorders. Anywhere from 11 to 20% of the population (depending on how it is assessed) will experience depression in their lifetime. Unlike the common cold, however, depression causes significant impairment in so many spheres of life—how individuals with depression think, feel, behave, and relate to others. As the partner of someone with depression, it certainly has a major impact on your life too.

Here is a breakdown of prevalence for particular depressive disorders:

- Major Depression: 10–20% of people over the course of a lifetime (about 7% in a given year)
- SAD: 10–20% of people who have major depression and about 3% of the general population
- Depression around pregnancy or postpartum: nearly 18%
- Persistent depressive disorder: about 1.3%
- Bipolar I disorder: around 1%
- Bipolar II: 0.4–1%
- Cyclothymia: <1%

The rates of depression in nonbinary and gender-diverse individuals are much higher, up to twice as common. This is likely due to a number of factors that include discrimination, harassment, stigmatization, and violence perpetrated toward gender nonconforming people in our society.

Is Depression "Normal" at My Partner's Age?

Depression can happen at any age, although the average age of onset is the early to mid-twenties. Depression is also a highly recurrent problem. Between 50 and 90% of individuals will experience additional episodes or have depression that is more chronic. For bipolar I and II, the typical age of someone receiving a diagnosis is around 25, although it can occur at any age.

Is Depression as Common in Men as in Women?

Depression tends to occur more often in women than in men with a consistent ratio of 2:1 that begins after the age of 12 years (prior to this age, rates of depression are roughly equal in females and males). The reasons for the differences are not entirely clear. One possible explanation is that women are more willing to open up about what they're feeling and acknowledge sadness whereas men may hide their depression or channel it in other ways such as alcohol or drug use. Research has not supported this idea. Men are, in fact, just as likely to admit to their depression as women. In addition, when men and women have the same levels of symptoms, they are equally likely to seek treatment.

Another explanation has been a biological one. As noted, differences in the rates of depression occur at the time of puberty, but there is a lot more going on than just hormonal shifts at this time. For example, young women experience more stress than young men. Stressful life events are strongly related to the onset of depression. In addition, this stress may work together with changes in estrogen and progesterone to make young women more sensitive to stress and, therefore, more vulnerable to depression.

Yet another important factor that differentiates women from men is rumination. Rumination (from the Latin word *ruminare,* meaning to chew over again) is when you think about or stew over something repeatedly. Research consistently shows that women ruminate more than men, which predicts the onset of depression following stress. Although this is an overgeneralization, women typically ruminate when something stressful happens and tend to think deeply about their social relationships: *What did I do? What did I say? Could I have said something different?* Men, on the other hand, stereotypically deal with stress by distracting themselves (playing video games, shooting pool, drinking, and the like).

Men and women are believed to have equal rates of bipolar disorder, although there is some evidence that this is climbing somewhat more in women. Men tend to have an earlier age of onset than women.

Is There a Specific Cause?

It's so easy to dwell on why your partner is depressed. Far too tempting to try to figure out the specific cause. The truth is that researchers have identified so many diverse factors that are associated with increased risk that it would be virtually impossible to determine what triggered your partner's depression. In general, research does not support the idea that any one risk factor is necessary and sufficient to cause depression. Instead, depression is caused by a combination of biological, psychological, and social factors. For some people, depression can be due to one factor more than another, but it is still most likely some combination.

Across multiple levels of scientific inquiry, research has identified at least 37 variables that could be considered causes of depression. Here are some of the potential causes:

- Numerous psychological factors, such as having an anxiety or substance use disorder, neuroticism (a personality trait where someone views the world as distressing, threatening, and unsafe)
- Negative thinking
- Rumination
- The way we learn to handle emotion
- Stressful life events
- Genetic influences
- Deficits in certain regions of the brain
- The body's stress management system (specifically the communication system between the hypothalamus, the pituitary gland and the adrenal gland of the endocrine system, or what is called the *HPA axis*)
- Loss
- Child sexual abuse
- Growing up with parents who didn't show a lot of warmth
- Having a parent die when you were a child

In most instances, there is a combination of some form of vulnerability with some form of stress. Someone with less psychological or biological vulnerability, for instance, would need more stress in their lives to tip them into depression, whereas someone who has more vulnerability would require less stress to trigger a depressive episode.

Here's the good news. Although there are many paths that lead to depression, there are also many pathways out, including effective, evidence-based psychological treatments, medication, and other options (see Chapter 3). There are also several strategies outlined in this book that you can apply to support your partner, cope with this yourself, and help improve your relationship. Let's get started.

2

Supporting Your Partner Effectively

Harper pulled up to the driveway and sat in her car for a few moments. She needed a couple minutes to decompress. She inhaled and exhaled slowly, bracing herself for what she might find at home. Harper predicted that her partner, Hiro, would be on the couch, still in pajamas or sweatpants, watching television. That made her feel bitter. She wanted to support Hiro, yet Harper felt ambivalent. She was sick of the caregiver role and tired of being the only one to keep everything running smoothly. Harper longed for a relationship that wasn't so one-sided.

When she got in the house, Harper walked to the den where she *knew* she would find Hiro. "Hey," she said. "Hey," Hiro mumbled back. "Did you eat today?" she asked. He shrugged. "Not really." That answer would typically make Harper rush to get something for Hiro to eat, but now it irritated her. She looked at him, slouched on the couch, unshaven, and appearing disheveled. Part of her wanted to hold him and tell Hiro that everything would be okay. Another part of her wanted to shake him.

You probably picked up this book because you're experiencing some of the same responses to your partner's depression as Harper. You may be struggling with balancing support for your partner with help for yourself and your relationship. You didn't ask to be a caregiver and might crave a more reciprocal relationship. Feelings like Harper's—ambivalence, worry, fatigue, resentment—are both valid and common among partners of individuals with depression.

Using some of the strategies outlined in this chapter (and throughout the book) will help you be the best support you can be. If you're worn out and frustrated, despite your love for your partner, being the best support you can be might understandably sound like a one-sided benefit. Please know that it's not. Yes, supporting your partner effectively will increase the odds that your partner's depression will improve. But it will also make your partner less likely to withdraw from you and isolate themself. You will be more able to deescalate conflict in conversations with your partner. You're likely to end up more satisfied in your relationship, and your relationship will have the best chance of healing, growing, and strengthening. Eventually, through your persistence, your partner may get to a point where they can reciprocate, and you will feel like you have a more rewarding relationship. You're probably reading this book because this is what you want.

The Importance of Social Support

Human beings are the most social of animals in the world, and our relationships contribute importantly to our physical and mental well-being. We are wired to be loved, to love, and to belong. Researchers have demonstrated, for example, that having strong social connections is a greater determinant of good health than smoking, high blood pressure, and obesity. When people feel well supported, they are healthier, have stronger immune systems, and, as a result, recover more quickly from physical illness. When someone is in physical pain, just seeing a picture of their supportive, romantic partner can reduce their levels of pain and decrease activity in areas of the brain that are associated with pain. In contrast, feeling lonely, isolated, or unsupported increases the risk of mortality and is associated with various health problems, including heart disease and stroke, high blood pressure, and chronic pain.

Social support also plays a major role in good mental health. Many studies suggest that feeling supported is beneficial to our mental health and can help us prevent, or recover from, various mental health problems. Being able to confide in others affords better stress management, lowers distress, and reduces the risk of experiencing depression. One study of more than 100,000 people tested the relationship between 106 modifiable risk factors and the odds of being depressed six to eight years later. The ability to confide in others rose to the top as *the number-one protective factor against depression.*

Social support involves feeling loved, valued, and having people you can turn to who will lend a hand when you are feeling down or need assistance. Unfortunately, individuals with clinical depression tend to feel less supported than people who don't experience mental health problems. This finding holds true in myriad studies across different nations, ages, and genders. When individuals with depression view their social support as inadequate, they experience more problems with depression and their chance of improvement worsens.

Being there for your partner when they are experiencing depression can help them function better and gives them the lift they need to carry on, improve, and even thrive. Feeling supported by you increases your partner's chance of feeling less stressed, experiencing more positive emotions, and having fewer symptoms of anxiety and depression.

The support you provide is critical not just for its potential benefits to your partner but also because you're likely the primary source of support for them. Partner support is relied on more frequently than support from family, friends, or other sources.

That undoubtedly sounds like a lot of pressure, especially when you add the fact that for social support to be effective it needs to be *perceived* as supportive by your partner. Otherwise, it generally won't be that helpful.

At this point you're probably thinking, *Oh great. Not only do I have to do all the giving, but I also have to make sure my attempts at support land with my partner! My partner perceives everything in a negative light, so how am I to know what will feel supportive?* Without really knowing what your partner is experiencing, how can you figure out what is working or not working? Do you use trial and error? Do you reach out, or back off? Do you give in to your partner's need to be alone, or try to connect? Do you provide solutions to their problems, or just let them work through it on their own?

You may want to encourage and provide support but are anxious about saying the wrong thing and setting off a cascade of negative feelings, frustration, and hurt. Perhaps you've tried many times, and nothing seems to change or, worse, you feel as though your partner doesn't want your support or neglects to follow through on any of your recommendations. Where do you begin?

Connect First

As much as we try to be a good support for our partners, we so easily flounder. That's often because we aren't always sure what to say. It's also because we jump to try to fix our partner's problems.

Isaiah came home after a long day at work and saw that Aiysha was feeling down. She had just gotten her performance evaluation from work, and it wasn't as positive as Aiysha was expecting. Isaiah tried to be as supportive as possible. Knowing that jumping in to try to fix things didn't work in the past, Isaiah tried hard to be supportive in a way that wasn't advice-giving. Unfortunately, it also didn't match what Aiysha needed. He said, "It will be okay. You'll be all right. I know you've worked hard for your promotion, but another opportunity will come along." Aiysha didn't feel heard. Instead, she felt as though Isaiah was trying to improve her feelings about the situation by shifting the way she thought about it. What she really needed was to be heard. Isaiah's intention was noble, but the impact was, well, not great.

The next day Aiysha met an acquaintance for coffee and mentioned her disappointment about the performance evaluation. This person, who Aiysha hardly knew, put her hand on Aiysha's and said, "I am so sorry. It's so difficult when you work so hard and don't get the recognition you deserve." Aiysha instantly felt heard, accepted, and understood.

Being understood, validated, and cared for is a constant human need. The need for other forms of support, like helping your partner reframe their circumstances or offering advice, varies depending on the situation and how well you can match your partner's needs.

Many years ago psychiatrist John Bowlby developed attachment theory, which has helped us understand not only the need to connect with our partner but also the predictions we make and the expectations we have in relationships. It has become the dominant model for understanding early social development and has a ton of research behind it.

The basic idea is that we develop an affectionate bond, called an *attachment,* early in life based on our contact with caregivers. If our caregivers were responsive to us and met our needs for security and safety, we developed a secure attachment, which meant that, as youngsters, we could explore the world around us and know that our caregivers would reliably be there for us (they provided a secure base). And we would expect future romantic and other relationships to function similarly.

Children whose primary caregivers didn't meet their needs or only met them inconsistently, develop an insecure attachment. For example, they may be anxiously attached, where they grow up believing they are not worthy of love and fear abandonment or rejection. These individuals may fear that future partners will reject them, and they may act clingy or hypervigilant to threats in their relationship. Someone who develops an avoidant attachment, on the other hand, likely had caregivers who were emotionally unavailable, didn't tolerate the expression of feelings, and raised the child to be emotionally tough and overly independent. Growing up, these individuals may not tolerate emotional or physical intimacy very well. Based on our attachment experiences, we tend to develop what's called an *internal working model.* This is basically our main way of viewing relationships—what we expect and what we perceive. This system becomes most activated when we are facing stress or adversity (for example, depression).

The main point is that there is a fundamental (nearly universal) need to connect, be heard, and be validated. We need our relationships to be secure and consistent for us. Your partner may not be there for you right now, at least not in the ways you would like them to be. That itself is depressing and disheartening. But when you are the best support you can be during this time, your partner is more likely to improve and start giving back to the relationship in the ways you need and desire. The second point is that by supporting our partners we can provide them with a safe haven (knowing that they can come to us for comfort) and a secure base (knowing that we will be there to support their goals and aspirations). As David Brooks noted in *How to Know a Person,* when we talk to someone, we're engaging in an "official" conversation and an "actual" conversation, the official conversation consisting of words and the topic being discussed and the actual one consisting of "the ebb and flow of underlying emotions being transmitted." The impact is that the person we are talking to either feels safer or more endangered with every comment.

When our partners are available, sensitive, and responsive to our needs, especially in a time of crisis, we have a sense of being securely attached. In contrast, when our partners are unresponsive, unavailable, or act insensitively, we are more likely to experience the attachment as insecure.

One way of providing support in a way that connects is to borrow from client-centered therapy, which highlights the importance of the therapist–client relationship (which decades of research have demonstrated is a necessary, although not sufficient, component of every effective psychological treatment). Client-centered therapy was developed by the famous psychologist Carl Rogers, who argued that people flourish when provided with the right conditions for growth. Just as a plant will naturally grow with adequate soil, water, and sunlight, your relationship with your partner will grow under certain conditions, including:

- ***Unconditional positive regard:*** Respecting and caring for your partner, their self-concept, and their feelings and accepting your partner for who they are.
- ***Genuineness:*** Being real, genuine, open, and authentic in your interactions with your partner.

- ***Empathy:*** Being attuned to your partner's feelings and beliefs and attempting to really understand and pinpoint your partner's experience and their inner world. Through empathy, you sense your partner's struggles and their thoughts and beliefs as though they were your own, without anger, fear, or confusion. With this clear sense of your partner's world, you can communicate understanding, including your awareness of what their experiences mean.

So, here's a good rule of thumb: always connect first. Provide messages to your partner that they are not alone in this. Messages that you understand and care. Messages that validate their experience. Messages of comfort, warmth, and simply being there: "I'm here for you. What can I do for you?" Then, if your partner wants other forms of support, provide those—but only with their permission.

TRY THIS: CONNECT FIRST

Experiment for a week or two with connecting first. When you are with your partner, try to relay messages that you are really there for them, that you are in this together. Show empathy. Express that you care. Practice with phrases like "I am here for you" or simply sit with your partner and demonstrate warmth and compassion and care. You will likely find that your partner feels more supported by these efforts than attempts to give them advice or provide information. Then, if they don't offer it up themself, ask them, "Are there other ways I can support you better?"

Connect or Cope?

One study looked at both connect and cope strategies. Connect strategies are a type of emotional support that focuses on helping your partner know that they aren't alone—that they are connected to you and valued by you. Cope strategies, on the other hand, focus on trying to help your partner feel better or to fix their problems: "I'll help you. I'll work to change how you feel. I'll try to provide information that may be useful. I'll support you in tangible ways." When researchers inquired about people's support preferences, they found that 81% of connect strategies were perceived as supportive whereas only 42% of cope strategies were believed to be helpful or supportive.

But if connect strategies are so helpful, why is it that we tend not to use them in our initial attempts to support our partners? Why, instead, do we try to cheer our partner up and provide hope that things will get better, as Isaiah did? Why is it that we offer informational support and advice about effective treatments or activities we have done that lift our own moods? How come we provide instrumental support that helps our partner deal with the demands of daily living, like booking or getting to appointments?

Because we don't *believe* that connect strategies are the most helpful. Validation of our partners seems less important to us than other types of support. We so desperately want to make our partners feel better *now.* We feel as though validation isn't providing the right "help" with the immediacy we need. Strangely, research demonstrates that even when supporters know that their partners want validation, they still lean toward trying to fix things.

Always connect first, then ask whether other support is wanted or needed.

Check Your "Fix-It Reflex"

Drs. William Miller and Stephen Rollnick developed motivational interviewing, an evidence-based treatment approach that helps people overcome ambivalence toward change. The approach was developed to help individuals overcome addictions and has since been expanded to other mental health problems where ambivalence might be an important feature. Rather than being characteristic of "addicted people," Miller and Rollnick postulated that the defensiveness and resistance to change in clients with substance use issues might be a result of how clients were being treated by their therapists. What they came to realize was that therapists tended to push for change and give advice, which backfired and was met with resistance when people were ambivalent about or not yet ready for change. The term they used to describe this tendency is the *righting reflex* (or the *fix-it reflex*).

TRY THIS: EXAMINING YOUR FIX-IT REFLEX

Have you ever had an experience where you were thinking of making changes in your life but felt kind of ambivalent? Perhaps you were contemplating losing weight, exercising more, or drinking less but weren't quite ready to put that ice cream away, sign up for a gym membership, or put aside that single-malt scotch. Now imagine that someone you love tries to persuade you to make this change, telling you all the reasons this change would be good for you and stressing how important it is. They might even list all the negative things that could happen if you don't make this change: how your appearance might get worse as you age, how your body won't recover as quickly from injury, how your cardiac health will diminish. In addition, they might highlight all the benefits that are in store for you if you did make this leap. They might even give you lots of advice about how you can go about making this change.

Take a few minutes to consider what your reaction would be to this well-intended act of persuasion and advice giving. How would you feel?

I do this exercise with my graduate class when we review motivational interviewing. Students in my class break off into pairs for about 10 minutes. One person acts as the persuader and the other as the person contemplating change. The responses are the same year after year. Students who were in the receiving end of getting advice felt angry, agitated, oppositional, and defensive. They felt as though they were not understood or heard; they felt discounted and invalidated; they felt overwhelmed, manipulated, ashamed, trapped, disengaged, uncomfortable, and resistant.

This is a normal human reaction to receiving unsolicited help and advice. We need to be careful to keep the "fix-it reflex" in check. Instead, we need to behold our partner and just be there for them rather than giving advice or trying to fix them.

Partners of individuals with depression can also fall into the trap of the "fix-it reflex." This is perfectly understandable. You want to make this right and may have very good ideas of the path your partner should take to improve their mood. Many people (men in particular) say they try to fix things for their partner whatever the problem is because they hate to see their loved one in pain and just want to help them eliminate it. The problem with this well-intentioned strategy is that it can lead to conflict, despair, and hurt.

Really Hear Your Partner

The fix-it reflex pushes us to act immediately, jump in to solve problems, and make things right for our partners when all they want is to connect, be validated, cared for, and heard. Unfortunately, as a society, we have become very poor at listening. Really listening. Part of the problem is that we are so enveloped in our own thoughts, deadlines, and objectives that we don't pause for long enough to simply be together.

I am very blessed to have grown up in a family that I adore. My parents modeled unconditional positive regard to me and demonstrated that love for each other. I also have a great relationship with my siblings and my nieces and nephew. When we are all together as a family, we often have a dinner (usually at my sister's place) and then play games or just sit around and chat. One evening, however, we were all on our devices, every one of us (including my father, who was no spring chicken). I was so amused and stunned by this that I took a photo.

In the age of instant gratification, we have learned to manage downtime by checking notifications and viewing our social media accounts. We have collectively lost the ability to really listen. When our partners are speaking, we are often thinking about what we are going to say next and neglect to really give them our full and undivided attention.

To listen well is a skill. It is more than just holding your tongue; it is active. Listening well is hard work. We must let go of our own needs, desires, and self-absorption and enter deeply into what our partner is experiencing and expressing. We need to forget ourselves and really attend to our partner. We can't simply pay lip service and feign attentiveness when what we are really doing is coming up with and rehearsing what we plan to say in return. When we prepare ourselves to respond, our ability to listen vanishes. We need to be there authentically. This is the essence of connecting—to really understand, value, and care for our partner.

Sometimes you may feel as though your partner is pushing you away. The natural inclination (largely for your own protection) is to withdraw and distance yourself. You might wonder why you even bother and proceed to build walls around yourself. What you really need to do is the opposite. You need to lean in. You need to forget about yourself and show your partner that you are there for them.

If you want some really excellent resources for learning how to listen well and connect with your partner, check out Brooks's *How to Know a Person* or Nichols and Straus's *The Lost Art of Listening.* These books masterfully describe how to fully attend and connect.

TRY THIS: REALLY LISTENING

The next time your partner is opening up to you or telling you about their day, just listen. Really try to immerse yourself in what they're saying. Don't rehearse what you want to say in return. Just listen. Try this out a few times and you might be surprised at your partner's response. It may take some time to get good at this, but by really listening to your partner—*really* listening—you will help them feel validated, cared for, and understood.

You Can't Read Minds

Research has demonstrated that there are different types of support: emotional, instrumental, informational, and cognitive. Emotional support involves being empathic, understanding, validating, and caring for your partner (the connect-first stuff we reviewed earlier). Instrumental support is helping your partner in tangible ways, doing things for them such as helping them fix a problem, cooking dinner, and meeting concrete needs. Informational support is providing suggestions and advice. Finally, cognitive support is trying to help your partner examine and reappraise themself or their circumstances from a different perspective. Of all these forms of support, emotional support is seen as most helpful. To reiterate, connect first, then ask whether other forms of support would be helpful.

A considerable amount of research has focused on the extent to which support provided matches what the recipient needs or desires. In general, high levels of support are related to lower distress and higher relationship satisfaction. However, as noted earlier in this chapter, good support needs to be tailored so that it is *perceived* as supportive.

What your partner requires at a particular time may differ from what they want on another occasion. From your perspective, you're being supportive. You may think that doing what you can—whether it is emotional, instrumental, informational, or cognitive—is what matters. But to be considered supportive and helpful to your partner, its quantity and quality must be what your partner wanted and needed. For example, at times and with every good intention, you may be providing too much or too little support for what your partner needs. This can negatively impact their mood and how satisfied they feel in the relationship. When you're better able to match the support you provide with your partner's needs, you're more likely to be seen as supportive, and the outcome will be more positive.

Sometimes we all project what we're feeling and assume that this is what our partner is going through. When we do this, we are likely to be inaccurate and unsupportive. Numerous studies have demonstrated that we don't predict well what people are thinking and feeling. When we base our support on what we think our partner needs, we're likely to make things worse. No one wants to hear advice that they didn't ask for. No one wants you to tell them that they should go to therapy or start a new regime of antidepressant medication. No one wants to be told that they should get outside of the house more or change their thinking. When we do this, we are only relaying the message that we don't really understand our partners and that their feelings and experiences are not valid.

You can't read your partner's mind. You don't have a crystal ball, nor do you have some superpower ability to accurately know what they are feeling and experiencing. Your aptitude for perceiving what others are thinking and feeling, in fact, typically sucks. One study found that married couples are accurate about their partners' thoughts and feelings only about 35% of the time at most. Which is why you need to ask your partner. We all need to listen. We need to get their take on the situation. From their mouths, in their words. Ironically, we tend to rely on our own experiences as a basis for making judgments about our partners when we have the least information. This is yet another reason to check with them.

Sometimes your partner may want advice, or assistance, or help reappraising their thinking. But here's the rule you should use; I am mentioning this a third time because I think it is *that* important: Rule 1, connect always. Rule 2, ask if they would like you to support them in other ways. If the answer is yes, then get the specifics of what they might truly be looking for.

It isn't all up to you. Your partner has an important role to play as well. They need to let you in rather than withdraw from you. As tough as it may be, they need to be able to express what they are going through and what support they need from you. They are most likely to do this when you connect first.

3

Becoming Informed about Treatments That Help

An important way to support your partner with depression is to learn about the many effective treatment options available. Treatment decisions will (or should) be made collaboratively by your partner's doctor and your partner, but you can be a good source of information if you take the time to inform yourself about what is available. This chapter will help you learn about what might work to ease your partner's symptoms of depression. Chapter 4 delves into how your partner can participate in treatment decisions.

As noted earlier (see Chapter 1), depression is caused by multiple factors. Because of this, searching for "the cause" of your partner's depression is likely to be futile and could lead you down the proverbial rabbit hole. Holding on to one explanation for your partner's depression may also have the unintended effect of limiting the treatment choices you and your partner think are available or appropriate.

Let's assume, for example, that you think your partner's depression is due to biological factors, perhaps their genetic makeup or the operation of brain chemicals (neurotransmitters, such as low levels of serotonin in the brain). A biological explanation for depression has some distinct advantages. For instance, it may make it easier for you to think that having depression is not your partner's fault. When you believe that your partner's depression is not controllable, you may tend to be more willing to help them and show sympathy. However, what does a biological explanation do to your perception of what treatments might be best? In this case, you might be inclined to consider only medical interventions, such as antidepressants, helpful. You might think that psychological treatments wouldn't be effective.

This would be an unfortunate conclusion for two main reasons. First, many psychological treatments are highly effective even for severe depression. As you'll learn later in this chapter, they also tend to have an important advantage, compared to medications, of reducing the risk of relapse and keeping people well. Second, the combination of psychotherapy and medication is often considered the optimal treatment choice for both depression and bipolar disorder.

This chapter highlights effective, evidence-based treatments for depression. Being informed about the various treatment options will ideally help you and your loved one find the most effective help. As they improve, your life and your relationship will get easier. We'll start by outlining some of the most effective psychological treatments, followed by discussing various medical interventions.

Psychological Treatments That Work

The approaches that have received the most extensive evaluations in randomized controlled trials (what researchers, through rigorous peer-reviewed research, consider the gold standard in scientific scrutiny) and meta-analyses (sophisticated ways of pooling together information from many randomized controlled trials to draw more definitive conclusions) are cognitive-behavioral therapy, behavioral activation, and interpersonal psychotherapy.

Cognitive-Behavioral Therapy

Of all the psychological treatments for depression, cognitive-behavioral therapy (CBT) has been the most well studied. CBT is based on decades of research showing that how we think about ourselves, our future, and those around us profoundly impacts how we behave and feel. CBT aims to help people shift their appraisals and beliefs from unhealthy and unhelpful to evidence-based and adaptive. By thinking differently, your partner will start to feel better and act differently. They will develop healthier beliefs about who they are and have a different outlook on their lives and their future. This will serve them better, but it will also make life easier for you.

A typical course of CBT for depression is 12 to 16 sessions long. The length of treatment may vary, however, depending on the severity of symptoms and whether there are other complicating factors, such as a coexisting medical or mental health problem. Many people notice significant improvement in as few as four to six sessions, but others may need longer.

Behavioral Work

As the name suggests, CBT offers a blend of both cognitive and behavioral strategies. Treatment often starts (especially in cases of more severe depression) with getting people more activated, an approach called *behavioral activation* (or BA). Behavioral activation can also be undertaken as a separate intervention, discussed on page 41. BA involves helping people gradually experience more pleasure in their lives and increase their motivation and ability to complete tasks that provide a sense of accomplishment. They also learn to approach rather than avoid. Although this isn't easy, especially at the beginning, people learn that if they act, even when they don't feel like doing something or can't seem to muster any energy, motivation and energy will eventually follow.

When I am lying in bed on a cold winter day, I don't feel like getting up and going to the gym. However, I tell myself, "Action comes before motivation." I need to act first and then motivation almost always catches up. If I push myself out of bed and drive to the gym, I'm motivated once I get there. On the other hand, if I wait for motivation to magically descend on me, I will probably just stay in bed, under my warm covers, 99% of the time.

Although the same principle works for depression, keep in mind that it's not that simple. There are many obstacles in the way when someone is feeling depressed. Sometimes even small tasks, like emptying the dishwasher or taking a shower, seem monumental. BA is a tall task in these circumstances. To make matters more complicated, your partner may criticize themself for being "lazy," "useless," or "weak" when physically or socially inactive. They may feel inadequate and helpless. In some situations they may also justify their avoidance by claiming that going out or being active wouldn't be fun or worth the effort. You've likely heard these excuses and been frustrated by them. This becomes a vicious cycle and makes them feel worse.

The more they withdraw from things, the more difficult it is to engage. Although avoidance results in misery, it seems easier (at least in the short term) to stay passive and socially isolated. Your partner may start to think they will never experience joy or satisfaction in their lives. They may also avoid things they previously enjoyed or valued because they predict that the activity won't be enjoyable or meaningful. The CBT therapist uses BA to help people think differently by acting differently—by approaching rather than avoiding; by breaking tasks into smaller, more manageable bits; by starting small and gradually moving forward, one step at a time. By behaving differently, we think differently and, by thinking differently, we feel better.

By becoming more activated, individuals with depression gradually start to feel more enjoyment and greater motivation. They begin to approach activities that provide them with a sense of accomplishment. They start to connect with others who give them a feeling of meaning and pleasure. This becomes reinforcing and serves to increase energy and lift depressed moods, which also helps to change their thinking. Through this process, for example, your partner may start to realize that they can do more than they thought. They may experience more pleasure or joy than they anticipated. They may start to realize that a big part of the problem has to do with how they're thinking about themself and the predictions they make.

Cognitive Work

Once people start to improve using behavioral strategies, therapy often quickly transitions to more cognitive work—learning to identify, test, and change negative thinking. There are several ways this is done. CBT therapists often start by demonstrating the power of our thoughts. They explain that it is not the situation in itself that impacts your response, but your belief. You might notice your partner feels bummed out and self-critical because they forgot to pick up milk from the grocery store. Although disappointing, it's not forgetting that produced their negative mood; it's the thought they had. If your partner thought, "I can't believe I forgot the milk. I forget everything. I am such a loser," they are likely to feel quite depressed and hopeless in this situation. However, if your partner thought, "I must have missed seeing it on the grocery list. Oh well, no use crying over 'forgotten milk.' No big deal. We all make mistakes. I'll pick some up tomorrow," they would have a completely different emotional response. The same situation, completely different responses. It's the thought that drives most of what we are feeling.

Let's say that you are walking down the hallway at work and your colleague passes right by you without acknowledging you. How would you feel? A little angry? Perhaps a bit sad? When you think of it, your colleague's not saying hello was not the *cause* of your emotional experience. Rather, it was the thought that you had about what happened that impacted your emotion. In this case you might have the thought "They don't like me" or "They intentionally dissed me." However, there could be several alternative explanations than the one that first came to mind. They may not have seen you. They might have been preoccupied and deep in thought. Maybe they received some bad news or were having a rough day.

I don't know about you, but when someone cuts me off in traffic, my automatic response is anger; not road rage anger but ticked off. To instill a sense of calm in these situations, I try to remind myself that this wasn't necessarily intentional and, even if it was, it's possible that something else is going on. Maybe they didn't see me. Perhaps they had some medical emergency and were trying to get to the hospital as quickly as possible. Even if I conclude that the driver was being a jerk, I still try to tell myself that I don't know what is happening in their lives and that there might be a valid reason they acted the way they did. Again, it's not the event (in this case being cut off in traffic) that leads to my anger but my thoughts. When I think differently, I am less angry. I am more able to cut them some slack and may even feel some compassion for them.

A key component of CBT also involves helping individuals track their thoughts and test them with evidence. When your partner is experiencing depression, their thinking is usually quite negative. They see themself through a negative lens that distorts their actual experiences. Not only that, but your partner is seldom aware of the negative thoughts that run through their minds. It becomes their default, automatic way of thinking. These thoughts just seem to pop up automatically without much attention paid to them. The problem with not keeping this barrage of negative thoughts in check is they aren't questioned or refuted. Instead, they are seen as truth, as fact, as valid, and continue to beat your partner down.

CBT helps to first understand moment-by-moment thoughts and test them out with evidence. Just like a researcher may have a hypothesis that they test out using an experiment, the therapist works to help people become scientists of their own thinking. Through this process, they learn to consider a thought as a hypothesis—as one possibility out of many alternatives—to be tested, rather than a done deal. By regularly examining and testing their beliefs, individuals in CBT learn to be more balanced and accurate in their thinking about themselves, others, and their future. This, in turn, usually helps lift depression.

Once someone begins learning this new way of thinking, the CBT therapist may also help them notice patterns in their thoughts (the usual culprits of negative thoughts that keep coming up). These frequent, negative thoughts often relate to more deeply held beliefs. For example, your partner may be invited out to join a friend for coffee but have fleeting thoughts that "They aren't really interested in getting together. They're just doing this because they feel sorry for me." These thoughts are likely related to a deeper belief about being unlovable. Alternatively, if your partner had an upcoming exam or assignment due at school and instantly thought "I don't have enough time to prepare. I can't handle this. I am going to fail. I'll bomb the assignment," they might have a deeper belief such as "I am incompetent."

These deeper beliefs commonly fall into three broad categories: being helpless, unlovable, or worthless. Some common beliefs that relate to being helpless include things like "I am incompetent," "I am weak," "I am a failure," "I'm a loser," "I'm defective," or "I am helpless." Unlovable beliefs tend to congregate around thoughts of being unlovable, unlikable, undesirable, unwanted, unattractive, or uncared for. Beliefs related to being worthless include "I am unacceptable," "I am evil," "I am rotten to the core," "I am bad," "I am a waste," "I am inadequate," and "I don't deserve to live." It's not your partner's fault that they have these beliefs. Often these beliefs are learned early in life for many different reasons. For example, perhaps your partner experienced some form of maltreatment as a child, either physical, sexual, or emotional abuse. Or perhaps their parents or caregivers were not very affectionate or available to them. Maybe they were bullied as a child on the playground or at school. Or it is possible they learned to think negatively about themself because of the messages they heard or acquired from others. Whatever the reason for their development, these beliefs are often so deep-seated that they're difficult to change. CBT can help to modify these deeper beliefs.

By learning to recognize these deeper beliefs, test them out with evidence, and modify them, people can make important changes to how they think, which improves depression and helps them remain depression free. By targeting these deeper beliefs, your partner will be able to experience less negative thinking overall. To illustrate, think about the moment-to-moment thoughts your partner has as leaves on a tree. You can pull one leaf off at a time, just like you can identify and change individual thoughts. You could even work hard to pull all the leaves off or grab a hedge trimmer to cut them all down in one fell swoop. However, the leaves will eventually come back. Unless you get to the root and cut off what is nourishing them, the leaves will continue to grow. Likewise, without getting to the root of your partner's negative thinking and cutting off the deeper beliefs that are nourishing them, negative, self-defeating thoughts will likely resurface and impact depression. By identifying and changing more entrenched negative beliefs, your partner's thoughts about who they are, how they view you and your relationship, and what the future holds will fundamentally shift. This different style of thinking will result in a new way of feeling and behaving—one that is free from the pit of depression.

CBT is highly collaborative and involves both the psychologist (or other licensed mental health professional) and your partner working together to discover negative thoughts and align them with evidence. People begin to view themselves and their experiences more objectively and compassionately, acknowledging that, although it is not their fault that they learned to think the way they do, there is hope that they can think differently in the future.

Behavioral Activation

Behavioral activation used within CBT as discussed above is somewhat different from behavioral activation as a stand-alone treatment. Used within CBT, behavioral activation focuses on addressing negative thought patterns that accompany avoidance and withdrawal. Research has demonstrated, however, that behavioral activation alone is also effective for the treatment of depression. In this approach, the focus is primarily on understanding the function of behavior (not on thinking) and trying to help clients understand that their mood is impacted by what precipitates and what follows what they do.

Individuals with depression often describe their lives as devoid of pleasure, gratification, feelings of accomplishment, and rewarding social interactions. This isn't surprising when you think about the symptoms of depression. When your partner is experiencing extreme fatigue, low motivation, concentration difficulties, and low energy, they tend to withdraw from many day-to-day activities. Who wouldn't want to just curl up in bed and shut the world out when you are feeling this way? However, the less you do, the less you feel like doing, and continued avoidance eventually creates a downward spiral toward more negative emotions and negative thinking.

Your partner might wake up feeling miserable. So, they press snooze multiple times or lie awake thinking about how awful they feel. Before they know it, the morning has passed, and they're still in bed. They may have thought this avoidance would improve their mood and energy, but it hasn't. Instead, it's depleted them. Have you ever had a day when you just sat there in front of the television binge-watching show after show on Netflix, Apple TV, or Disney+? What happens to your energy when you do this? I'm guessing it drops like a lead balloon. Although I don't do this often, when I end up watching a lot of television on a particular day, I feel worse. My back gets sore from the lack of movement, my head feels cloudy, and I feel more tired than when I started.

Avoidance becomes a vicious cycle. After lying in bed all morning, your partner will likely feel less energy and motivation. In addition, they will probably start to beat themself up mentally for wasting the day. This negative thinking will then make your partner feel worse (more tired, more depressed) which then contributes to more avoidance. Because of this avoidance, your partner is not experiencing opportunities that might be pleasurable, meaningful, or connects them with you or others—three things are key in improving moods.

Behavioral activation helps people with depression reengage and improve their mood by modifying their avoidance, withdrawal, and inactivity. Although it's not quite as simple as I'm describing, the main idea is that we need to act differently to feel differently—that depression can be treated effectively when an individual learns to act from the outside-in rather than inside-out. In other words, instead of allowing a mood to dictate what you do or don't do, you push yourself to act in ways that are antidepressant, regardless of how you are feeling. By doing so, mood, energy, motivation, and life satisfaction eventually improve, and depression starts to lift.

More about this in Chapter 5 when we review strategies to help your partner reengage and reduce avoidance.

Interpersonal Psychotherapy

Interpersonal psychotherapy (IPT) focuses on the idea that depression results from difficulties people have in their everyday relationships and that, by improving the life problem, you can relieve symptoms of depression.

IPT is a highly focused intervention that typically occurs over 12 to 16 weekly sessions. At the beginning of treatment, the therapist works collaboratively to find out what interpersonal issues are impacting depression. These issues fall into four main categories: (1) relationship disputes, (2) role transitions, (3) grief, and (4) interpersonal deficits. To find out which interpersonal issue is most pertinent, the therapist would take time to review how your partner is functioning in daily social interactions, find out about close relationships in their life, and understand relationship patterns and expectations.

Relationship disputes refer to the conflicts that people have in their romantic relationships, with family members or with friends or other social contacts. These conflicts may arise because of problems communicating with others or because of unrealistic expectations. For example, an individual may be dealing with relationships that are overly hostile or where there is verbal or physical abuse. There may be conflicting loyalties within the family. There may be arguments over the lack of intimacy in the relationship. Someone may feel as though their loved one doesn't reciprocate affection or do their fair share of the work in the relationship. After the specific problem is identified, the IPT therapist works with them to create a plan of action for dealing with it. The therapist helps the individual identify the source of misunderstanding, see whether this pattern is evident in other relationships as well, and learn strategies for communicating and solving problems more effectively. Sometimes this might involve reviewing a recent incident that occurred and trying to respond differently.

Carmela mentioned to her therapist that she and her partner had a fight after dinner on Wednesday evening. She concluded from this interaction that "my partner never listens to me." This thought resulted in Carmela's feeling angry, hopeless, and depressed. In this case, the IPT therapist might try to analyze the situation to find out what wasn't working quite right in the communication: what was Carmela saying that was not being relayed in a productive way? How was this interfering with the relationship or causing conflict? How did her partner, Shannon, respond? How did Carmela respond in turn? From this, Carmela was able to recognize that she started the conversation being critical of Shannon. Instead of overgeneralizing and assuming Shannon never listens, Carmela might come to realize that her partner shut off when she was critical. When Carmela could understand that Shannon wasn't listening to her *because* she had started the conversation in a critical way, Carmela could change her view of the situation from "Shannon never listens to me" to "Shannon doesn't listen to me when I am critical of her." Although Carmela may still feel bad, and it could take time and negotiation with Shannon to work through these issues, this insight could provide Carmela with more hope that things could change and a new strategy to try out when interacting with Shannon.

Another interpersonal problem focused on in IPT has to do with role transitions. These refer to life changes that are difficult to adapt to, such as the loss of a job, retirement, "empty nest syndrome," buying a new house, financial gain or loss, marriage, divorce, the diagnosis of a chronic medical condition, and so on. In these cases the IPT therapist helps develop a more well-rounded, realistic perception of the change, grieve the loss of the old role and express these emotions, and see the new role in a more constructive, positive light. In addition to helping someone see things differently, the IPT therapist will also work to help them learn new skills or refine their expectations so that they can adapt more easily to the change.

When someone is experiencing grief or loss, the IPT therapist helps them process their emotions surrounding the loss, ensure that there is adequate support around them, and, in some cases, develop strategies for forming new relationships that might help buffer the impact of the loss.

Finally, interpersonal deficits become the focus of therapy if an individual reports that they have a low number of friends or poor quality of social relationships. Sometimes problems arise because of the way one communicates with others. For example, some people with depression can rely too heavily on other people or might be highly sensitive in social situations, taking everything personally. They might fear being scrutinized or evaluated. Others might have an interpersonal style where they respond to others in a hostile way. It is also possible that someone lacks connections with others because they don't have the skills needed to develop or maintain healthy relationships. In these instances, the IPT therapist helps the person develop new skills for interacting with others, identify and change styles of communicating that interfere with close and satisfying relationships, reduce their social isolation, and increase their social network.

All three of these approaches—CBT, behavioral activation, and IPT—tend to focus on the here and now. There is no archeological dig of the past. This doesn't mean that the past isn't important, but reflects the idea that greater therapeutic change can take place when you target the thoughts, behaviors, and interpersonal problems that are affecting depression right now.

Psychological Treatments for Bipolar Disorder

Although medication is the most effective form of treatment for bipolar disorder, the addition of psychological treatments improves outcome and reduces the risk of relapse. Three main approaches have demonstrated strong efficacy in research trials: cognitive therapy, family-focused therapy, and interpersonal and social rhythm therapy.

Cognitive therapy for bipolar disorder is very similar to CBT for depression as described earlier. However, much of the focus is also on helping individuals with bipolar disorder learn how to regulate their sleep and day-to-day routines, identify early triggers of manic symptoms, and best adhere to their medication prescriptions—all of which can reduce the risk of relapse.

Family-focused therapy helps people, and their loved ones, learn about bipolar disorder and enhance communication and problem solving. They learn about triggers of mania and depression, understand the risk of future episodes, accept the necessity of being on mood-stabilizing medication, distinguish the individual's personality from their disorder, learn to cope with stress that may trigger additional episodes, and improve family and couple interactions.

Interpersonal and social rhythm therapy is based on the idea that interruptions in one's daily routine (such as not getting enough sleep) and conflicts in a relationship can increase the risk of relapse in bipolar disorder. This treatment helps people maintain a consistent sleep schedule, manage stress, and improve overall relationships.

Each of these treatments have been shown to work equally well and to improve outcomes better than medication alone. So, if your partner is experiencing bipolar disorder, they may really benefit from one of these psychological interventions as an adjunct to medication.

Biological Treatment Options

In addition to psychological interventions, numerous medical treatment options are available. The most well known is antidepressant medication. Antidepressant medication tends to work as well as psychotherapy, and in many cases combining the two may provide the most help. When depression is severe, physicians often prescribe antidepressants because they may be quicker to provide relief. Keep in mind, however, that CBT and some other psychological treatments are also effective for treating severe depression.

Pharmaceutical companies are very powerful and have a ton of money to advertise and promote their products. Billions of dollars are spent every year to target consumers directly. These ads are plastered all over television, in magazines, online, and in social media. Although these ads may educate the public about treatment options and encourage a discussion with their doctors, the real purpose is to encourage patients to make requests of their physicians for certain brands of prescription drugs, which may lead to biased or unnecessary prescribing.

Medications certainly have their place in the effective treatment of depression. However, myths about depression are also spread on advertising and social media. One myth is that depression is simply a problem with our biology. In other words, when someone is depressed, there is something wrong with their brain chemistry. Let's assume your partner is prescribed a medication like Prozac (fluoxetine), which increases the amount of a neurotransmitter called *serotonin* in the brain. Their mood improves, and the conclusion might be that depression is a result of low serotonin in the brain. However, the logic behind this is not always sound. For instance, just because you can relieve a headache by popping a couple of Tylenol capsules doesn't mean that the headache was due to a lack of acetaminophen.

For decades, the "chemical imbalance" theory of depression has prevailed and resulted in a massive increase in the use of antidepressants. This makes sense: if you are told that your brain chemistry is out of whack, then it seems reasonable to take a medication that helps to balance and stabilize this. Yet recent research suggests that this theory is not well supported by scientific evidence. The truth is that we don't really know what antidepressants are doing to the brain, and continuing to promote the idea that depression is caused by low serotonin, norepinephrine, dopamine, or some other chemical imbalance, is misinformation. In his book *Anatomy of an Epidemic,* Robert Whitaker provides a brilliant and scathing review of the flawed science behind psychiatric drugs and argues that the problem of depression has only gotten worse during the modern drug era.

A related myth is that just as someone who is diabetic needs to take insulin, someone with depression needs to be on an antidepressant. This is simply not true, and researchers have demonstrated that even severe depression can be treated effectively with CBT and other evidence-based psychological approaches.

Medication seems to benefit individuals who are suffering from moderate to severe or chronic depression. They provide little or no help at all in milder forms of depression. In those cases, it would be better to see a psychologist or other licensed mental health professional, sign up for an online program that teaches evidence-based ways to manage depression, or consult a good self-help book that is grounded in science. Ask your health care provider for some recommendations about these resources. In the case of individuals with bipolar disorder, mood-stabilizing medications are necessary; psychological treatments can help improve functioning and serve as an adjunct to medication.

For most people with depression, antidepressants work as well as psychotherapy. Although medication can provide relief of sadness and other symptoms, no pill will cure depression. In fact, people often experience a relapse or recurrence of their depression once they stop taking medication. This has led medical practitioners to recommend that individuals continue their medication regime for a period of at least six to nine months (and sometimes up to a year or two) after their depression has improved to reduce the risk that depression will return (an approach called *continuance medication*). In contrast, those who are treated with evidence-based psychological treatments like CBT are more likely than those treated with medication alone to remain well because this approach trains them to think and behave differently, skills that can last a lifetime.

If your partner is interested in taking antidepressant medication, the first step would be to consult with their family doctor or get a referral to see a psychiatrist. Often this requires a healthy dose of patience and a period of trial and error. Your partner may have to try different medications to see what works best for them. When prescribing a medication, physicians aim for what's called the *therapeutic window*. This is the optimal balance where your partner will experience a relief of symptoms without having too many side effects from the medication. It takes at least four to six weeks to see if a medication is working. Once this therapeutic window is accomplished, there may also need to be other tweaks in the prescription over time. For example, physicians will often add another medication to augment the effects of the initial prescription. The good news is that there are many options available. Your family doctor or psychiatrist has 31 different antidepressants to choose from, 17 of which are considered first-line treatments because of their safety profile and because the evidence has supported their efficacy in randomized clinical trials.

Types of Antidepressants

Let's take a brief look at some of the antidepressants available as of the publication of this book. The selective serotonin reuptake inhibitors (SSRIs) are recommended as the first medications to try because they tend to have the fewest side effects (these can sometimes include insomnia, nausea, feeling sleepy, or problems with sexual functioning), are generally safe to prescribe (they are not lethal if someone overdoses on them), and they are easy to take (it usually involves taking only one pill a day). Although I won't provide a review of the proposed neurobiological mechanisms of action, these medications are believed to work by increasing the availability of serotonin in the brain. Celexa (citalopram), Lexapro (escitalopram), Luvox (fluvoxamine), Paxil (paroxetine), Prozac (fluoxetine), and Zoloft (sertraline) are commonly prescribed SSRIs.

Tricyclic antidepressants, developed in the 1950s, are the oldest class of medications for the treatment of depression. These medications are believed to work by increasing norepinephrine (and, to some extent, serotonin) in the brain. These include medications such as Anafranil (clomipramine), Elavil (amitriptyline), Norpramin (desipramine), Pamelor (nortriptyline), Sinequan (doxepin), and Tofranil (imipramine). A host of side effects accompany these medications, including dry mouth, blurry vision, weight gain, sleepiness, constipation, difficult urinating, dizziness, and abnormal heart rhythms. They also tend to be lethal if used in overdose.

Another class of medications, used less often because of severe side effects, are the monoamine oxidase inhibitors. These medications work to reduce an enzyme (monoamine oxidase) from breaking down the neurotransmitters dopamine, norepinephrine, and serotonin, thereby making more of these available for electrical and chemical activity in the brain. These medications not only have dangerous side effects but also require avoiding certain foods that can raise blood pressure when taken together with these medications.

Several other classes of medications have come on the scene more recently, like the serotonin-norepinephrine reuptake inhibitors. These include medications such as Cymbalta (duloxetine), Desyrel (trazodone), Effexor (venlafaxine), Pristiq (desvenlafaxine), and Remeron (mirtazapine). These are also recommended as first-line interventions.

Generally, between 50 and 70% of individuals respond to antidepressant medications. No one class of medications works better than another, so the decision of which medication to go on would involve a discussion with your family doctor or psychiatrist, who will make a recommendation based on several factors, including potential side effects, medical history, symptoms of depression, cost, family history, and so on.

Medications for Bipolar Disorder

In contrast to major depression, which is caused by multiple psychological, social, and biological factors, bipolar disorder is quite genetically loaded. For example, if one identical twin has depression, the chances are only about 40% that the other sibling will experience depression. However, if an identical twin has bipolar disorder, the odds are much higher, around 72%. As a result, medication is extremely important in the treatment of bipolar disorder. Bipolar disorder is typically treated using lithium, anticonvulsants, or antipsychotic medications. Although we don't really know specifically how lithium works, it has been shown to help stabilize mood swings. Common side effects include significant weight gain, dehydration, acne, thinning of the hair, and hand tremors. People also need to be monitored closely on this medication because it can affect thyroid and kidney functioning. Anticonvulsant and antipsychotic medications can also be prescribed either alone or in combination with lithium to control mania.

Phototherapy for Seasonal Affective Disorder

As mentioned in Chapter 1, seasonal affective disorder is a type of depression that affects individuals during the winter months, where there are low periods of light. Phototherapy uses a special lamp to provide doses of light (~10,000 lux of white light) that help improve an individual's wake and sleep cycle and improve depressed mood. The procedure involves sitting in front of a special light that mimics sunlight anywhere from 30 minutes to two hours a day.

Other Biological Interventions

Other interventions are used when several other approaches have been attempted and people are still not getting the symptom relief they need.

Electroconvulsive therapy (ECT) involves inducing a brief (typically 25 seconds) seizure by applying an electrical current to a person's brain two to three times a week for a total of 6–12 sessions. Although ECT continues to conjure up negative images from the past (remember the film *One Flew over the Cuckoo's Nest*?), modern-day ECT is well monitored and conducted in a way that minimizes physical risk. For example, blood pressure is monitored throughout, mouth guards are worn to prevent injury to a patient's tongue or teeth, and a general anesthetic and muscle relaxant are administered so that people don't convulse during the procedure. ECT is quite effective for difficult-to-treat depression (60 to 80% of patients will experience remission) and used for depression that is really severe and life-threatening.

Transcranial magnetic stimulation (TMS) is another approach that involves placing an electromagnetic coil on an individual's scalp, creating a magnetic pulse that causes small electric currents in the brain. The procedure is painless and lasts about 20 to 40 minutes a day, several times a week for four to six weeks. How TMS works to improve depression is not well understood, but it is believed that the magnetic pulses increase activity in parts of the brain.

Between 50 and 60% of people who have not benefited from medications respond to TMS. For a third of these individuals, the symptoms seem to go away completely, although not permanently. Most people feel better for several months and up to about a year. As with medications, the risk of relapse is high for both ECT and TMS and often requires scheduling future treatments.

How Well Do These Treatments Work?

Generally speaking, the recommended course of treatment for mild to moderate depression includes psychotherapy (ideally CBT, behavioral activation, or IPT) initially without medication. If depression is mild, your partner can also try a number of great self-help books or online interventions that are available.

For more moderate to severe depression, either high-intensity psychological intervention (usually CBT, behavioral activation, or IPT) or antidepressant medication is recommended. A combination of high-intensity psychological intervention and antidepressant medication may also be most appropriate for moderate to severe depression in individuals who have had poor response to one treatment alone or have responded well to combination treatment in the past.

The research demonstrates that CBT is equally effective as medication for the treatment of depression (even when it is severe). The same appears to be true for behavioral activation and IPT. In fact, CBT, behavioral activation, and IPT are all strongly recommended by various expert treatment guidelines as a first line of treatment. CBT also has an enduring effect, compared to medication, in preventing the risk of relapse. Individuals who are treated with CBT experience less than half the relapse rates of those treated with medication alone. And it is at least as effective as continuance mediation. Research also supports the long-term benefits of behavioral activation and IPT for the reduction of relapse risk. In contrast, antidepressant medications appear to suppress symptoms of depression only for as long as they are being taken. Once medication is discontinued, many people experience a recurrence of their symptoms.

If you made it through this chapter, you now have a lot of information about current effective treatments for depression. Many options are available, so don't lose hope. The treatment(s) that your partner selects should be those that are based on the best evidence available. But there are other factors to consider as well. In the next chapter, we will work through how to help your partner make this selection. I also discuss how to broach the topic of treatment with your partner and how to best support them through this process.

4

Encouraging Treatment

What you've read so far has laid important groundwork for supporting your partner, yourself, and your relationship. You've built an understanding of how depression works as well as what can help alleviate debilitating symptoms. You've learned the importance of connecting first and resisting the urge to jump in and fix things. Knowledge is power, and this valuable information will help you support your partner's efforts to get effective treatment.

In this chapter, we'll move toward more action-oriented strategies to help your partner feel better. Importantly, they can also help you. As you see your partner start to feel better and communicate more, reengaging in a way that you may not have seen in a long time, both of you will gain hope that the burden of depression is lifting. You'll begin to feel more optimistic that you can get your partner back and the relationship can heal.

Before moving on, I'd like to pause for a moment to check in with you—in the same way that I regularly check in with patients to get a sense of how their symptoms are improving. At pivotal points like this, I usually do a more formal review with questionnaires that help me assess whether we're heading in the right direction or need to shift course a bit. But here I'd like to offer you an opportunity to just reflect on whether you (and your partner) are ready for the next steps in this chapter.

TRY THIS: ARE YOU READY TO MOVE INTO ACTION?

How are you managing as you work through this book? Are you struggling to apply some of the strategies reviewed so far? What are your thoughts? Do you feel inspired to dive in and forge ahead, or are you feeling overwhelmed or hopeless? Some of the support and communication strategies in Chapter 2 may require considerable practice before you begin to see results. One option might be to put the book down for now and focus your efforts on connecting first. There is no magic solution for managing your partner's depression, and it can take some time for these skills to develop or for your partner to be receptive to them. Maybe much more time than you anticipated.

Trust the process. You'll get there. If you've worked at some of the connect-first strategies and feel as though you are ready for next steps, go ahead and read on.

This chapter focuses on helping you discuss what you've observed and encouraging your partner to get help. We'll also address how to discuss depression with your partner's primary care provider, how to choose a psychologist or other mental health professional, and how you can assist with treatment.

Barriers to Seeking Treatment

Depression impacts more than 350 million people worldwide. Sadly, since the COVID-19 pandemic, the rates of depression have increased even further. Although depression is common, and effective psychological and medical treatments are available, most people don't receive the help they need either because they aren't interested in seeking treatment or they have difficulty accessing it. In fact, just one in three individuals with severe depression and one in five with moderate depression seek help from a mental health professional each year.

Before speaking to your partner about getting professional help, it's important to be aware of some of the obstacles that might get in the way. Your partner may hesitate to pursue treatment for any of these reasons:

- A tendency to minimize the severity of their problems
- Difficulties with telling others about their troubles
- Fear of stigma and embarrassment
- Lack of time for treatment
- Negative ideas about treatment
- Lack of knowledge about available treatments
- Lack of health insurance or other financial constraints

Don had always prided himself on being strong and self-sufficient. He was the person others leaned on when things were chaotic, grounded and calm even when facing a lot of stress. So when he lost interest in things he used to love and felt down and mentally flat, he didn't sweat it too much. Don assumed he was overtired or dealing with too much pressure at work.

Bianca noticed that something wasn't quite right. At first she let it ride out, assuming everyone has off days. But Don's low mood and lethargy continued for a couple of months. He regularly stayed up too late and woke up exhausted. He declined friends' invitations and seemed more withdrawn. Bianca, who had a fantastic sense of humor, used to make Don laugh all the time—but now he hardly ever laughed. Even producing a smile seemed forced. He wasn't himself.

Bianca finally asked, "Have you thought about talking to someone?" Don shook his head. "Nah, I don't need therapy. It's nothing—probably just stress. I can handle this on my own."

Bianca didn't press the subject at first. She figured he knew himself. The longer this went on, however, the more Bianca worried about Don and the more their relationship became strained. Every time she brought up the topic, Don dismissed it. He always had a reason: "I don't have time. We can't afford it. This is something I should be able to manage on my own. Getting help for 'mental problems' means you're weak."

Like Don, many people with depression don't seek care because they fail to recognize their symptoms as signs of depression or they believe they should be able to pull through on their own.

Another huge barrier to seeking help can be your resistance as the partner. You may believe you should be able to handle your partner's depression on your own, or that they should be able to get through it without any professional help at all. Maybe you find yourself thinking, *If I just helped them change their diet, exercise more, or get better sleep, their depression might improve.* Or: *If I help them keep busy or talk about it more, they might climb out of this.* All of these are reasonable and generally helpful strategies, but getting the right help is crucial, especially for more severe depression. Most people with clinical depression need treatment to recover.

Addressing Your Partner's Concerns and Misconceptions

Working through your partner's apprehensions with them can help them accept the treatment they need—as long as your goal is to be as caring and nonjudgmental as possible. I know this is not an easy feat, especially when you've been through so much yourself, but it's an approach that will pay off for you in the end. It's so easy to think that telling our partners what to do is supportive or even a way of showing love. Although the intention might be good, it can be perceived as judgment.

Your partner might think their problems aren't serious enough to warrant professional help. We often downplay the severity of our problems or think that time heals all wounds. Let's be honest: time doesn't heal all wounds, and that's certainly the case with depression. Although depression can sometimes get better on its own (something we call "spontaneous remission"), it's a recurrent problem and, over time, future episodes can be triggered by less and less stress. Getting the right treatment can not only help your partner get better more quickly but can minimize the odds that depression will return.

Like Don, your partner might think that seeing a therapist is a sign of weakness, that they are a failure, or that they *should* be able to get through this on their own. In contrast, realizing the need for help and seeking it is usually a sign of strength. If you broke your leg and were unable to walk without assistance, this wouldn't be a sign of weakness but instead an indication that you need support. A crutch is just that—a temporary support. It doesn't mean that you'll need it forever or that you'll never be able to walk independently again. The same is true for therapy for depression.

With some gentle questioning, you might ask your partner how they would view a friend or loved one if *they* decided to get professional help. My guess is that they wouldn't see it as a weakness or a failure. Individuals with depression often exhibit this kind of double standard. They hold themself to a higher bar than everyone else: "It's okay for *others* to seek help, but *I* should be able to cope on my own."

Another common perception is that getting help is too expensive. In the United States and Canada, psychotherapy is typically paid for out-of-pocket or through private insurance, which often provides only limited coverage for mental health. Government-supported health care can include therapy, but waitlists to see a specialist like a psychologist or a psychiatrist are often long. The thought of adding expenses like these to your other obligations might be overwhelming. This may require some careful thought and discussion with your partner.

Could you think of it as an investment, one that has the potential to pay off in dividends for both of you? The typical course of psychotherapy for depression is not cheap; an adequate dose of treatment can cost a few thousand dollars or more. You don't want to throw caution to the wind, but you might want to weigh the pros and cons of getting help versus maintaining the status quo. Approaches like CBT and behavioral activation are cost-effective in the long run (even more so than medication) because they not only treat the depressive episode but also reduce the risk that depression will return.

There are likely options for readers who are strapped for cash. For instance, it may be possible to get help through an Employee Assistance Program or access free mental health support. Many therapists also offer a sliding scale for people who are not able to pay full price. So, inquire if this represents your situation. Local universities or hospitals also have training programs in which you may be able to access therapy for free or at a reduced rate. I am currently working with a colleague at my university to offer free therapy to help train some of our doctoral clinical psychology students. Sessions are closely monitored and supervised by licensed psychologists, but therapy is delivered free of charge by doctoral trainees.

Online therapy options may also be less expensive. In this case, the research generally shows that therapist-assisted online treatments (where an expert can be contacted periodically to check in and deal with questions or motivational issues) produce better outcomes than self-directed online programs (where you learn the material and go through the strategies on your own). Alternatively, you can try exploring self-help books, particularly if your partner's depression is less severe. In this case, be careful to do your homework and ensure that what is being offered is based on scientific findings and not empty promises. There are a lot of great self-help books out there, but there is also a lot of garbage. One book I highly recommend is *Mind over Mood,* written by two experts in CBT, Dennis Greenberger and Christine Padesky.

Your partner might also believe that you, their friends, or family will be able to help them as much as therapy can. There's no doubt that a strong support system is important for our mental health and that friends and family can help us through many difficult challenges. However, you can only do so much to support your partner, and your resources are not infinite. It can easily reach a tipping point where you aren't able to provide enough assistance because you're exhausted and feeling the strain of your partner's depression on your relationship. In addition, you don't have the formal training or knowledge required to deliver therapy. Working with a mental health professional who has the expertise needed to best treat depression can be invaluable. In these instances, it's beneficial to share your perspective with your partner and encourage them to get the right help from people who are well trained to deliver evidence-based treatments.

When your partner is ready, share what you've learned so far about effective ways to treat depression. Give them a sense of how you think therapy can help and how their depression is affecting you and the relationship.

TRY THIS: TALKING ABOUT GETTING HELP

Take time to prepare for a discussion with your partner. Think about what they are going through, from their perspective, and how they might respond to your suggestion of seeking help. Put yourself in their shoes. Will they be open to the idea? Might they be offended? Could they minimize their problems? Are they going to react with shame or embarrassment?

Before you have this conversation, come up with a game plan. Nothing written in stone—you want to be flexible in your response—but a general plan for some ways you might respond so your partner won't get their back up.

You probably know your partner better than anyone. So take a moment to reflect. Consider some of the beliefs your partner could have that interfere with their openness to consider professional help. Be prepared to respond in a caring and validating way. Then figure out the optimal timing to bring up your concerns. When the moment is right (not perfect, but right) share what you've observed and why it's concerning you.

Be gentle and don't push too much, but have an honest discussion with them about what you have noticed and why you're concerned. Tell your loved one how you see depression impacting them. Be candid about how it's affecting you and your relationship but try to avoid the blame game. Instead, point out the specific behaviors you've observed—that you have noticed they've been crying more, losing interest in things, or withdrawing from you and others.

Your loved one may try to minimize their experience or chalk it up to recent stress, but be persistent: "I understand that you have been going through a lot lately, but I have noticed you haven't been yourself for some time now. You seem to have lost interest in most things and aren't as animated as you used to be. Are you willing to talk about it?"

Although it might be difficult to discuss, don't avoid raising concerns about your partner's well-being. It's easy to get distracted or come up with excuses, but avoidance only helps in the short term. It generally results in greater pain down the road. When your partner is feeling sad, you might think, *I don't want to upset them now.* Conversely, when they are having a good day, you might say to yourself, *They are finally feeling more upbeat. I don't want to rock the boat.* Don't wait for the perfect moment. It'll never come. You could end up repeatedly making excuses, and avoiding the topic won't help either of you. Talking this through is essential for your partner's well-being, for your own sanity, and for the health of your relationship.

Don't Push Too Much (although Sometimes You Need To)

People respond in different ways to the suggestion of getting professional help. If your partner agrees with you and sees things the way you do, great. You are ready to start talking about treatment options and sharing what you've learned. If your loved one doesn't see it that way, it can be frustrating, and tough to recognize that there may be valid reasons they're feeling this way. You may feel powerless, sad, or even angry that they are minimizing their symptoms or refusing to get help. These emotions are understandable. Although you may think that being confrontational can be motivating for your partner, it usually backfires. Confrontation can work in some instances but usually decreases motivation to seek help in individuals with depression. Be patient. Think of it as planting the initial seed. Give your partner some time. Let the idea germinate.

Remember the discussion in Chapter 2 of the tendency to want to jump in and fix things? Be on guard for that and resist the urge. Your timing may not be your partner's timing. For sure, there are times when you may need to be more direct or get to the point where an ultimatum is warranted. Hopefully you aren't there yet. Initially approach this as a dance with your partner, where you lead them through the steps without their really noticing, not as a wrestling match, where you push and they pull. Unfortunately, the more severe the depression, the less inclined people are to view help-seeking in a favorable light. So, give it time. Try to help your partner disclose what they are going through by asking questions. Listen with compassion and try to understand their reservations. Hopefully your partner will come around once they recognize that your motives are noble and that you are truly there to stand with them through this.

As difficult as it may be for you to accept, seeking treatment is their choice. Let your partner know that you'll support them whatever decision they make but that you genuinely believe getting help is an important step forward for them and for your relationship. If your partner's depression is more serious or they may be at risk of harming themself or others, you'll obviously need to act more quickly. In this case you should contact a health care provider, mental health provider, or emergency medical services. These issues are discussed in Chapter 7.

It's also important to know when to stop. You can't force your partner to get help. It is a decision that they need to make. And they may not be ready yet. Persuading may only push them away and generate hurt and pain for both of you. Give them space and time and accept that they may never be ready for therapy. You may not agree with it, but the drive for change must come from them.

Meeting with Your Partner's Primary Care Provider

If your partner is agreeable to talking about depression with their primary care provider, they may want to come up with a plan. Offer to have a discussion about what they want to tell their provider and whether they have specific questions in mind. Once you're there, it's easy to forget what you want to say or ask, so think about writing down some of these thoughts and questions before you go. It may also be helpful to list the symptoms your partner is experiencing and specific ways depression is interfering with their life. Although the medical practitioner will no doubt share their perspective on what the best treatment options might be, it would be advantageous to figure out ahead of time whether your partner is interested in taking antidepressant medication, would like a referral for CBT (or some other evidence-based therapy for depression), or a combination. Remember, there are advantages and disadvantages to each, so make sure your partner understands these trade-offs. If not, that's okay too. Your partner will hear some recommendations from your primary care provider.

Although they may want to go alone, you could offer to attend the appointment with your partner to provide support and possibly add information about what you've observed. During the appointment, make sure that you're prepared for your partner to be in the driver's seat. Empower and encourage them to be honest about their experiences and express any hesitations or preferences they have about treatment. Your partner (or you if that's okay with your partner) should ask about the range of treatment options available and make sure you both understand the advantages and disadvantages of each, including how helpful the treatment might be, how quickly you might expect depression to improve, side effects, and so on. Your partner should be sure to ask as many questions as needed to feel confident and comfortable with your decision.

Meeting with a Psychologist (or Other Mental Health Provider)

The primary care provider may refer your partner to a psychologist or other mental health professional who specializes in evidence-based practice. A referral typically isn't necessary unless you are seeing someone through the public health care system (at a hospital, community, or primary care site). Many mental health professionals in private practice also accept self-referrals. It would be important to check with your partner's insurance provider if you have extended health benefits to see a mental health provider in private practice. Ask about the amount of coverage and whether the insurance company requires a referral to cover the full or partial costs.

Just like meeting with a primary care provider, it's helpful to prepare ahead of time for the first appointment with the mental health provider by writing down your observations. What symptoms have you and your partner noticed? How long has the depression been going on? Are there times when your partner's mood worsens or improves? What patterns have you noticed? In what ways is depression impacting your partner's life? What are some helpful or unhelpful coping strategies they use (such as exercise or alcohol)? You might also want to come up with a list of questions, such as what your partner can expect in treatment.

The first appointment is usually focused on conducting a thorough assessment to help the psychologist or other mental health provider get a clear sense of what your partner is going through. They will ask several questions about symptoms, how long they've lasted, and when their depression began. They will ask about whether this is the first time your partner has experienced depression or if there have been other episodes. The mental health professional will also ask about past and current treatments your partner has tried to deal with depression and the extent to which they have been helpful. Your partner's family medical and psychological history will be reviewed. Your partner can also expect to be asked about their use of alcohol, cannabis, or other prescribed or unprescribed drugs. There will be questions about basic lifestyle like sleep, diet, exercise, and leisure activities. Your partner will also likely be asked about their educational background, developmental milestones, and social supports.

Your loved one may be asked to complete questionnaires about their symptoms or some of the negative thoughts they are experiencing. This gives the provider an idea of how severe their depression may be. The purpose of this assessment interview is to understand what your partner is going through and figure out how they can best help. Toward the end of the assessment, the psychologist or other mental health professional will present their view of the situation, likely share a diagnosis, and develop a treatment plan. They should also outline the pros and cons of different treatment options. Your partner should feel free to ask any questions so that they can make an informed decision about whether they want to work with the provider and understand how treatment would proceed.

Finding a Therapist

Choosing the right therapist with the right skills is important. It's a decision that will significantly affect the odds that your partner's depression will improve and that they'll stay well. This can be a daunting and unsettling task. Who should they reach out to? Should they see a psychologist, psychiatrist, social worker, or counselor? How will we know who might be the best option?

Your partner will want to make sure they're working with someone who understands them and demonstrates compassion and empathy. Considerable research demonstrates that the connection people feel with their therapist (the therapeutic relationship) is critical for making the strides needed to improve. Although necessary, the therapeutic relationship is not sufficient for change.

You and your partner should view the therapeutic relationship as the foundation of your partner's treatment. Like the foundation of a house, if it has cracks or is unstable, the entire edifice can falter. However, a foundation also doesn't make a house. You need the framing and the roof, the insulation, and the drywall. You need the proper plumbing and electrical work. Similarly, the therapy relationship, although hugely important in treatment success, is only part of the equation. You and your partner also want to ensure that the therapy provider has the right credentials, that they are intimately familiar with the research, and that they are trained to provide evidence-based care.

It's your right to ask questions about your provider's training, background, and approach:

- What is your professional background and degree?
- How familiar are you with treating depression?
- What treatment(s) do you use to help people with depression?
- What would the general treatment plan look like?
- How do you keep track of progress in therapy?
- Is my partner able to attend sessions or play some kind of role in treatment?

A good therapist will be open to these questions and provide as much information as your partner needs to feel comfortable working with them. They might encourage your involvement (especially at the beginning) so that you can understand how to best support your partner in making these important changes.

Several professional paths can lead to a career in psychotherapy. However, the provision of therapy itself is not regulated. Basically, anyone can "hang up a shingle" and claim to do therapy. The term *psychotherapist* is generic and, although there are exceptions, typically does not require any training or certification. At a bare minimum, it's important to make sure that the provider you choose is properly trained to do evidence-based therapy, has a license to practice, and is registered with a professional body. Licensing is intended to protect the public by ensuring that the professional meets the standards of practice and has sufficient training. It also provides a mechanism for disciplinary action should that ever be necessary.

Although psychologists are the professionals most likely to use evidence-based approaches like CBT, behavioral activation, or interpersonal psychotherapy, some other professionals (such as psychiatrists, clinical social workers) are sometimes also trained in these modalities.

The PhD (Doctor of Philosophy) or PsyD (Doctor of Psychology) is the minimum requirement to become a psychologist in most jurisdictions. Psychologists receive a bachelor's degree in psychology and do six to eight years of postgraduate training that involves coursework, research, practicum placements in various clinical settings, a full year of residency and a postdoctoral year, in which they do clinical work, under supervision. They must also complete professional exams to be licensed. They are highly trained and qualified to diagnose and treat depression and other mental health conditions. Psychologists are also well trained in assessment, and are the only mental health professionals qualified to administer and interpret many psychological and sophisticated cognitive tests.

Psychiatrists have a medical degree and then complete a three- to five-year residency in psychiatry, which provides hands-on training (mainly in medical management, such as prescribing medications) followed by a clinical fellowship. They focus primarily on prescribing medications and are well trained in the types of medications that impact mental health conditions. Not all psychiatrists are well trained in providing psychotherapy, although some are. Traditionally, psychiatrists view depression from a biological model, meaning they believe antidepressants or other medical interventions are critical to the treatment of depression. However, some psychiatrists understand and value psychological interventions and are trained to deliver evidence-based psychotherapy.

Most social workers complete a four-year undergraduate degree in social work followed by a two-year master's degree. They also do fieldwork in a variety of settings, such as mental health clinics and child and family service agencies.

The choice of which professional to work with will come down to many factors, including how severe your partner's depression is, your partner's preference for medication, psychotherapy, or both, access to seeing someone in the health care system, and your financial situation. If your partner's depression is severe, the first line of treatment should involve a combination of medication and an evidence-based psychological treatment (CBT, behavioral activation, or interpersonal psychotherapy, see Chapter 3). Your partner should feel comfortable with the person they decide to work with, and that person should be well trained and experienced to treat depression. My belief is that seeing a psychologist would be the best choice for evidence-based psychotherapy. For medication, you would want to see your primary care provider or get a referral for a psychiatrist. Although sometimes more difficult to get access to, psychiatrists are specialists in prescribing medications used to treat mental health disorders (psychotropic medications) and may offer more than a primary care provider if your partner's depression is more severe or complex.

Take time to familiarize yourself and your partner with the different psychological treatments covered in Chapter 3. This will equip you to know what to expect from a particular treatment. If your therapist states that they know their treatment works based *solely* on their experience, this should raise a red flag. You want a therapist who is relying on the research evidence and knows the scientific literature. They should also be able to talk about how effective the treatment is and what its limits are. The provider should also be able to develop a formulation about your partner's depression—a theory about what may be causing the depression and why it's continuing. They should be able to explain to your partner how this formulation leads to the treatment plan. You can even suggest a trial period for therapy. This will give your partner an opportunity to see how they feel working with a particular professional and give them a sense of how therapy can be helpful. Regardless of your choice, if a particular treatment provider doesn't work out, don't give up. It's okay to cut ties and find another professional to work with.

Facilitating Treatment

There is not a lot of research on the benefits of using partners to facilitate treatment outcomes. What is out there suggests that it can be helpful, although possibly no better than therapy alone. However, there may be other benefits including increased empathy and understanding, decreasing blame, and demonstrating that you are on the same team and that depression is a "we" problem and not something your partner has to grapple with on their own. It can also help to create a stronger bond between the two of you by promoting more open and honest communication.

If you joining some therapy sessions is agreeable to your partner and their mental health professional, this can be a great opportunity to better learn how depression affects your partner. It can also help you learn strategies to nudge your partner toward change and encourage them to stick with the treatment plans.

Therapy sessions are typically only 50 minutes once a week. That means that there are 10,030 minutes outside of the therapy session that can either promote or hinder your partner's progress. Your support can help your partner make the most of this time. For instance, you might be able to work with your partner as they complete different components of the treatment (therapy homework assignments), such as assisting with behavioral activation or with helping them monitor, test, and change negative thoughts.

Lots to think about when encouraging your partner to seek treatment. I hope this information helps you feel more comfortable and confident in how to proceed. In the next two chapters we'll review strategies for helping your partner do things that are antidepressant and change their thinking. Let's move on.

5

Helping Your Partner Engage in Antidepressant Behavior

You may feel as if your partner isn't willing (or able) to do anything. So it would be only natural to wonder how you're supposed to help your loved one engage in antidepressant behavior. Watching the person you love living in a world that seems to get smaller and smaller can be frustrating and disheartening. You want to help your partner but may be losing hope that you can.

Jocelyn has been with John for nearly a decade. John has experienced depression off and on over the past five years. Two years ago, John said he needed more space and decided to move into the spare room. Jocelyn allowed him to create that space because she was trying to be supportive and show she cared. But now she doesn't know what to do. As her eyes welled up with tears, she said, "You're still in the spare room! Because you haven't dealt with things, you need more space, and the space you have doesn't feel big enough. You feel small because you live in one tiny room in the house! You feel unwelcome, but you have created that for yourself. And everyone else is allowing you to create that space because it's one of the few things you've asked for." Instead of helping the couple move *toward* each other, they had started drifting apart. Living in the spare room became the new normal.

You might feel as though you're getting sucked into the same void and your world is also shrinking. You haven't been able to get together with family or friends for far too long. Plans are constantly canceled. All the work around the house—from cleaning, to cooking, to paying bills, to mowing the lawn (or shoveling snow if you live in cooler regions)—falls on your lap. There doesn't seem to be any joy in the relationship. It's all work and no play. You are exhausted trying to keep up.

What if there were strategies you could try to make things better for you—some tools that will empower you to help your partner be more motivated, energized, and engaged? Helping your partner reengage bit by bit just might start to expand their world, making your partner feel better, and that, in turn, might make you feel better. You'll find such strategies in this chapter.

Here's how it works: antidepressant behavior, like getting more active, can improve your partner's depression symptoms. As that happens, your partner's thinking will also shift. Your partner will begin to see a glimmer of hope and become less negative. Your partner's mood will also change, and you might see more expressions of joy in them. You may notice more zip in their step. You will see them doing more, which will help you experience more pleasurable activities and lift some of the heavy load you've been carrying. When you start to feel better and respond positively, your partner's behavioral changes will be reinforced, and that will help you both keep the momentum going. It's a step-by-step process and, although it may seem like an impossible task right now, you will get there.

How Avoidance Zaps Energy and Contributes to Depression

Your partner's experience of depression has likely included a downward spiral of withdrawal and avoidance. It might feel as though they aren't doing anything and are deliberately avoiding everything. Let's look at how avoidance keeps the depression cycle going.

Although a disheartening experience for you, and a difficult trap for them, avoidance makes a lot of sense. Being depressed leaves people with low energy, a pervasive loss of interest in things they used to enjoy, and a marked drop in motivation. Concentration difficulties interfere with the ability to attend to things that previously produced a sense of accomplishment or pleasure. Your loved one may be tired all the time, feeling as though every movement takes a special kind of effort. When they feel like this, the natural inclination is to pull back from their usual responsibilities, avoid being active, withdraw from others, hibernate, and literally shut out the world.

The problem is that avoidance helps people feel better only in the short term. Over the long run it depletes energy and makes depression worse. It's not fair that you need to jump in and suddenly take on new roles as encourager, coach, and manager or that you are simultaneously responsible for your partner's well-being and household obligations.

Avoidance is like adding fuel to a fire. It quickly becomes reinforcing and self-perpetuating. The less your partner does, the less they feel they can do, and they start to spiral downward (see the diagram on page 67). It's an easy trap to fall into. Your partner might have spent the morning in bed, binge-watched streaming shows, or just sat there, practically immobile. This lack of activity results in even lower energy. Then your partner starts to beat themself up mentally for being so passive. Meanwhile, you are standing on the sidelines feeling helpless, discouraged, and maybe even aggravated, wondering what to do.

The good news is that it's possible to turn the downward spiral around. It can take time, but with some concerted effort and gradually putting one foot in front of the other, your partner can shift the spiral upward. They will begin to approach things they've been avoiding and start to do things that give them a sense of pleasure and feelings of accomplishment. By doing this deliberately (and eventually more frequently), your loved one will regain some energy and motivation. Their mood will improve, and negative thinking will dissipate. This, in turn, will give them hope that their depression can get better. Approaching—rather than avoiding—will become reinforcing, allowing them to slowly take on more responsibilities and experience more pleasurable activities. It is a gradual process, but there is good research evidence that behavioral activation is effective for depression.

How Behavioral Activation Works

Do you remember the Nike slogan "Just Do It"? Behavioral activation, introduced earlier in this book, works similarly. Often when people are depressed, their thinking operates from the inside out: "I feel miserable, so I am not going to join my friend for coffee today" or "I have no energy; I'll leave the dishes for another day." Individuals with depression use how they are feeling in the moment as the gauge for whether they should act and when. Does this help? Well, kind of—at least in the short term. It's always easier to avoid. However, your partner will never benefit from recognizing that pushing themself to go out or do some small task might have a positive effect on their mood, an effect that will increase the chances that they will do more down the road. Doing more will increase your partner's confidence. They will experience a sense of accomplishment. They will feel more energy. They will begin to experience pleasure again. Doing activities that are (or used to be) enjoyable will improve your partner's mood. It may not happen right away, and it may take every fiber of their being to muster the energy necessary, but one way out of depression

The Downward Spiral in Depression

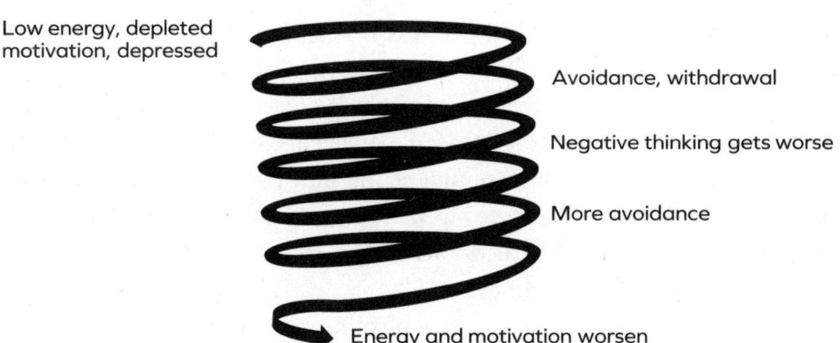

is to approach more and avoid less. Odds are that, over time, they will feel less tired, think more clearly, and start to feel more confident. Chances are good that they will begin to experience pleasure again. They may also begin to reconnect with you and with family and friends, which can also help to turn depression around.

To do this, your partner needs to learn to operate from the outside in: to act according to planned activities and set goals rather than acting on how they are feeling: "Although I don't feel like meeting my friend for coffee, I know that doing things that are antidepressant will help me down the road. I need to act even though I don't feel like it." Action comes before motivation. Once you start, motivation usually follows.

This is where you come in. It's a tough balancing act, because you don't want to nag, argue with your partner, or make them feel guilty. You also don't want to reinforce myths that depression means your partner is lazy or just isn't working hard enough. However, some gentle encouragement to try this out might lead to success. Your partner might eventually be willing to approach this with you systematically and deliberately. This won't be easy, especially at the beginning. Stick with it. Be patient. You and your partner will likely be thankful you did.

How to Help Your Partner Engage in Behavioral Activation

Taking a systematic, step-by-step approach can make behavioral activation easier for your partner to adopt.

1. Share What You Know

You might want to begin by taking time to have a conversation with your partner about how avoidance obliterates our energy and contributes to depression and how behavioral activation can help. As discussed in Chapter 2, start by connecting first. Validate what your partner is going through. Take time to listen. Help them see that you understand how trapped they feel; that you know they would like to do more but their symptoms are holding them back. Relay your understanding of how awful they feel and that it makes perfect sense they feel the need to withdraw.

You might mention that depression is like a beast that is sitting on your partner, sucking the life out of them (think of a Dementor from *Harry Potter*), suffocating them, making them feel tired, sad, and hopeless, telling them things that feed their depression: "You won't enjoy it. It's not worth the effort. You're no good at it. This is too difficult. It won't be fun like it used to be. Why bother? Nothing seems to matter." One way to counter the beast is to stop feeding it. When we avoid our problems and withdraw from activities, we tend to have more negative thoughts, feel worse, and have less energy and motivation. If you're so inclined, you could even draw a personalized version of the downward spiral.

When we do things that are pleasurable and meaningful, connect more with others, and become active, depression tends to improve, as shown in the diagram on page 69. Although it may take some time and work, your partner will feel better when more active. Emphasize that you are there for your partner and relay the idea that together you can start to confront the beast of depression.

2. Start Small

Your partner may not easily buy into the idea that behavioral activation is going to benefit them. So, you may instead want to begin by more subtly encouraging them to engage. You will likely have to give it ongoing effort. It can take time for people to experience pleasure or to gain a sense of accomplishment when depressed. Once they've seen the benefits of engaging in activities that are pleasurable or meaningful, however, they may be more open to hearing the rationale behind why behavioral activation helps reduce depression (and they will have some initial evidence that it works). You know your partner better than anyone, so you make the call.

Steve loved to go to the gym and kept encouraging Lisa to join him: "You know, activity is really good for you!" Lisa felt invalidated and protested, "How

How Behavioral Activation Helps Lift Depression

Do more of what you value
Pleasure
Accomplishments
Connections
Feel better about yourself
Joy
Confidence
Positive mood
Meaning
Motivation

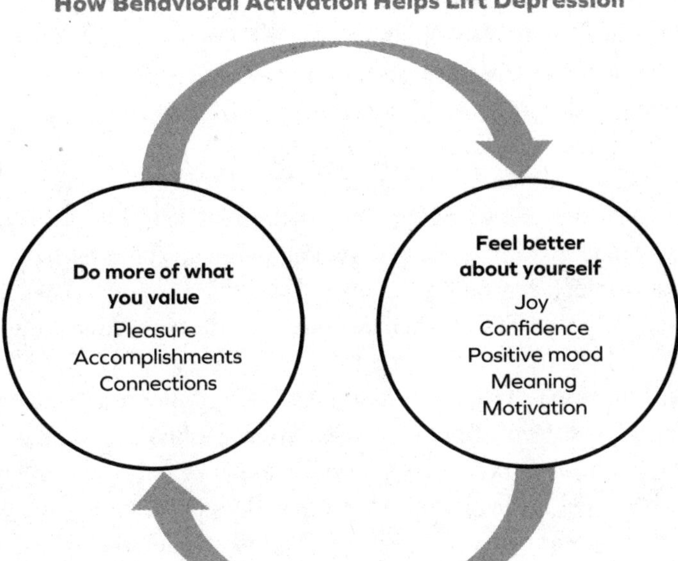

can you tell me to get active when I'm feeling absolutely crummy?" Trying to be more sympathetic, Steve later approached it differently. "How about we go for a short walk this evening?" Not surprisingly, Lisa was more receptive to that idea. Steve learned that he could encourage Lisa by breaking bigger tasks into smaller components. One day, instead of proposing that they go for a swim, Steve suggested that he and Lisa just sit by their pool and dip their feet in the cool water. With his gentle persistence, Lisa started to see the benefits of being more active and was willing to work with Steve to develop a plan they could work on together.

Sometimes the way you phrase things can help make your partner more receptive. For instance, instead of suggesting that doing something more engaging will help them feel better, you could say, "I'm kind of tired of watching television. Why don't we read together instead?" Rather than preaching the benefits of getting some fresh air, you could try, "It's a beautiful day today. How about we have supper outside tonight?" or "Why don't we drive to Dairy Queen and have a dipped cone at the picnic table?" Encouraging your partner to do something with you might make the activity less overwhelming and more enjoyable for both of you.

Capitalizing on things that your partner may already be doing might also help give you a bit of an in. For example, if your partner is driving home from an appointment, you could offer to meet them somewhere for a walk or a coffee. If they have finally made it out of the bedroom, you could invite them to join the family for supper or suggest playing a board game.

You might also want to give some thought to activities your partner used to enjoy but hasn't done for some time because of depression. Jake, for example, used to be so vibrant and energetic. That's what initially attracted Lydia to him. Jake used to enjoy reading James Patterson books, hiking up the trails near their home, working out, and playing guitar in the evenings. Early in their relationship, Jake would serenade Lydia with classic rock tunes that they both loved. Lydia's eyes lit up when he sang to her. But over time, things began to change.

The shift wasn't dramatic at first. Jake's energy started to wane, and the spark he once had slowly dimmed. At first Lydia attributed it to the stress Jake was experiencing at work. But days turned into weeks and weeks into months. Jake barely picked up his guitar anymore and stopped going for hikes and working out. He was halfway through the latest Patterson thriller when he no longer seemed able to concentrate, and the book sat untouched for months on their coffee table. Lydia missed seeing him play his music and the hikes they used to take together when they would talk, laugh, reminisce about the past, and dream about the future.

Now Jake seemed to have lost interest in everything. Lydia knew she couldn't "fix" Jake or tell him to "snap out of it"—she had to meet him where he was, gently and patiently. Lydia started with something small. Rather than suggesting that Jake pick up his guitar and sing to her, Lydia recommended going for a short walk outside. Jake was hesitant at first but eventually complied. The walk resulted in a small victory that didn't demand too much of Jake. The next day, Lydia suggested a little more—a quick walk to the nearby coffee shop. It took some time, but Jake eventually started to respond. Lydia continued to encourage Jake to do something, no matter how little it was, and she was consistent in her effort. They started walking a little farther and spending time in the park by the river watching the geese and goslings. The walks became part of their routine. One evening Lydia tentatively handed him the guitar. She wasn't pushy. She simply said, "Just strum if you feel like it. No pressure. I miss hearing you play, that's all." Although Jake managed to strum only a few chords, he returned to his guitar more regularly over the next few weeks. Lydia knew it wasn't the solution—there was a lot more work to do—but it gave her a glimmer of hope. Step by step, they would add more activities that brought Jake pleasure and gave him a sense of accomplishment.

TRY THIS: START BY SUGGESTING SOME ACTIVITIES YOUR PARTNER USED TO ENJOY

Take time for a little reflection: What did your partner enjoy that they are no longer doing? Coming up with activities where there is already some buy-in may help kick-start the process. Think about some things that you could begin to include in your partner's routine, even if that means starting with showering every morning and getting up at a regular time. Then start to introduce some ideas that your partner can do on their own or you can do together as a couple. The box on pages 72–73 provides a list of examples. Don't give up if your partner declines your offer. Start small and slowly progress toward more activation.

There are literally hundreds of activities you and your partner can try. Everyone has their own tastes and preferences, so see what might pique your partner's interest most, which may very well be something your partner once pursued eagerly. At least at first, it might be helpful to find some activities that you can do together as a couple.

You may have already tried this many times and found your partner constantly declines to participate. If so, try reminding your partner that you're attempting to help them feel better and that this is important for them, for you, and for your relationship: "I know that you don't feel like doing this and that it seems like more effort than it's worth, but I want us to work together as partners to tackle this. Would you be willing to give this a try?"

3. Take an Activity Inventory

Another important strategy, one that will need some buy-in from your partner, is to monitor activity. Just as it does for every retail store, taking an inventory of what's selling and what you need more or less of can provide a lot of useful information.

In a sense you're "selling" activity to your partner, and it can be helpful to both of you to know what to stock their days with and what to avoid. Your partner can take an inventory of the activities they engage in during the week, rating how these activities have affected their moods. Are the activities that seem to produce a low mood monotonous, ruminative, asocial, or unrewarding? If so, remove those from your list. An activity inventory can

Some Pleasurable Activities You May Try with Your Partner

- Reading a good book
- Listening to music
- Taking a hot bath with candles
- Baking cookies or a cake
- Doing a puzzle
- Painting or drawing
- Watching a movie or TV series
- Playing a board game or card game
- Organizing a relaxing corner for yourself
- Watching a sunrise or sunset from your window
- Dancing around to your favorite songs
- Doing a craft project
- Aromatherapy with essential oils
- Playing video games
- Cooking a new recipe
- Doing a face mask or skincare routine
- Knitting or crocheting
- Sipping tea or coffee in a cozy setting
- A new hobby (for example, calligraphy, photography, small engine repair)
- Meditating or practicing mindfulness
- Decluttering your space for a fresh vibe
- Creating a scrapbook or photo album
- Playing with a pet
- Doing a guided workout or yoga session
- Listening to a podcast
- Giving yourself a manicure or pedicure
- Journaling your thoughts
- Creating a playlist
- Watching a documentary on a subject you're curious about
- Learning a new language
- Observing nature
- Making a meal with friends or family
- Doing a home spa day
- An online dance class or tutorial
- Making a bucket list
- Creating a garden or indoor plant setup
- Having a virtual hangout with friends
- Watching a live stream of a concert or event
- Organizing a photo shoot at home
- Watching nostalgic childhood cartoons or shows
- Playing with puzzles on an app or online
- Going on a hike
- Stargazing on a clear night
- Going to the beach and feeling the waves
- Riding a bike around the park or neighborhood
- Having a picnic in the park
- Cross-country skiing
- Taking a walk in a botanical garden
- Traveling to a new city or town for the weekend
- Walking barefoot in the grass or sand
- Going for a scenic drive
- Spending the day at an amusement park

- Visiting a local farmers' market
- Going for a swim in a pool or lake
- Going kayaking or canoeing
- Doing a photography walk
- Horseback riding
- Exploring a national park
- Birdwatching in a peaceful area
- Going on a road trip to a nearby destination
- Ice skating or inline skating
- Paddleboarding or wakeboarding
- Attending an outdoor concert or festival
- Watching wildlife in a reserve or sanctuary
- Swinging at a playground
- Going to a botanical garden or greenhouse
- Playing frisbee or catch with a friend
- Doing a scenic bike tour
- Reading while sitting by a lake or river
- Picking fresh fruit or flowers at a farm
- Taking a leisurely walk through your neighborhood
- Sexual intimacy

also help point out what activities help lift their mood and help you understand why. Are they pleasurable for your partner? Do they provide a sense of accomplishment? If so, look for other activities that do the same. We know that depression is related to a lack of reinforcement. Reinforce what makes your partner feel better by restocking their schedule with antidepressant activities.

TRY THIS: ACTIVITY LOG

One way to begin taking an inventory is to create a basic calendar that has the days of the week at the top and the hours in the day on the side (see the form on page 74 for an example). For each waking hour of the day, your partner would record what they are doing. For each time slot, your partner would also record their mood from 0 to 10, where 0 is feeling very depressed and 10 represents feeling very good.

Your partner doesn't need to get too detailed in their recording, but it's helpful to record what they're doing on the activity inventory (even if some things don't seem relevant or important to them). The main goal at this stage is to find out how your partner's mood changes when they're engaged in different activities.

Although creating an activity inventory can help you see the whole week in a couple of pages, there are other ways to do this if you find them more convenient. For example, your partner could just record (on a pad of paper or their note-taking app on their phone) what they're up to for each hour of the day and how they're feeling. There are also a variety of activity tracking apps available online. They also have the option of monitoring morning, afternoon, and evening times if hourly recordings are too much at first.

Regardless of how your partner decides to track their activity, completing an activity inventory for at least one week can be helpful, although you may want to extend this if the week was not typical (for example, you went away on vacation, or you had guests in from out of town, or your partner was ill). You and your partner may also want to continue the activity inventory for a longer period of time if you find it helpful. Often when we start monitoring—whether it's drinking, smoking, exercise, diet, or mood—our behavior tends to improve.

A warning and word of advice: One objective in completing the activity inventory is simply to help your partner understand what they are doing throughout the week and how that impacts their mood. It is super important to stress to your partner that there is no judgment on your part and try to ensure that they don't judge themself either. It is too easy to complete the activity inventory and think, "Geez, I am doing nothing! I am so lazy, incompetent, and inept." Unfortunately, this can be a common reaction. Some people might

Sample Activity Inventory

	Mon.	Tues.	Weds.	Thurs.	Fri.	Sat.	Sun.
6–7 A.M.							
7–8 A.M.							
8–9 A.M.							
9–10 A.M.							
and so forth							

even feel more stuck when they do the activity inventory and may become consumed with guilt or shame.

You can help your partner by encouraging them to suspend judgment for now: “This is the nature of depression, but there is hope. The past isn't as important as deciding what to do now. What matters more than what you've been doing is what you try to do now. Let's work together to help you put one foot in front of the other so that you can feel better.”

Your partner may start comparing where they are now with what they used to be capable of: *I used to do so much more. I used to have energy. I used to be productive. Now I'm practically immobile. I am pathetic.* An analogy may be useful. If your partner fell off a roof and broke both legs, it would take time to get back to normal. They would first need to rest and heal. Then they would need to do some physical therapy to regain the strength in the muscles that have atrophied from being in a cast for so long. They might need to be supported physically as they grasp the parallel bars and slowly drag their feet forward one inch at a time. Once they regain more strength, they might move along the parallel bars quicker, requiring less support over time. Then they might be able to walk without assistance and work on regaining a sense of balance. Eventually, with a lot of hard work, they may begin to jog or even run. It would do them little good to lie on the hospital bed lamenting that they can't do anything and comparing themself to people who run long distances. This only makes them feel demoralized. Likewise, it won't help them to reflect on what they could do before the depression. Instead, encourage them to focus on step-by-step improvement rather than reflecting on the past.

4. Look for Patterns

Once your partner has monitored their activity for a week, they can start to examine the activity inventory for patterns. Can the two of you find some connections between your partner's activities and their mood? Did their mood change at all over the course of the week? What were they doing?

The idea here is for your partner to try to figure out how their behavior impacts their mood:

- What are the worst times of the day for them?
- What days of the week are harder?
- What was your partner doing (or not doing) when their mood was worse?

- When was their mood a bit better?
- What were they up to when their mood was better?
- What things might your loved one be avoiding?

This information gives you some ideas of where your partner could start to make some changes.

Hopefully your partner will be open to having you review the activity inventory with them. Two heads are often better than one, and they may find it helpful to have you involved. It is also possible that they will want to do this on their own. If that's the case, give them space and let them explore. Unfortunately, your partner may not want to do this at all. *You* may not even want to do this. If that is the case, don't sweat it. There will be other ways you can help them get more active. You may find, however, that systematically encouraging more and more activity may help your partner come around and start to see the benefits.

Take a look at the sample activity inventory on pages 77–78. It was completed by Nicole, who had been in a relationship with Keith since they met in high school 13 years ago. Nicole had experienced bouts of depression off and on for the last few years, but this most recent episode was the worst, and Nicole needed to take a leave from work.

As shown in this example, Nicole's mood was pretty bad throughout the day. Because Keith had been helping Nicole get a little more active, especially when he got home from work, Nicole was receptive to having Keith help her review the activity inventory. They noticed that Nicole felt her lowest when she was more passive, spending time in bed, watching television, or playing games on her phone. Conversely, Nicole's mood was better when she was doing something active like walking the dog, helping to cook supper, or doing some small chores around the house. Nicole's mood was best when she was not only doing something active but also connecting with others. Nicole seemed to perk up most when she and Keith joined some friends at an escape room. Although Nicole didn't feel as though she contributed to solving the puzzles as much as others, it was enjoyable to get out and her friends even managed to evoke a few laughs. Other times when Nicole's mood improved were when she joined a friend for a walk, went to her parents' for supper, or had an intimate brunch with Keith.

They both knew that it would take time for Nicole's mood to improve further (the best her mood got this week was a 6 out of 10, and that was a rare occurrence), but they agreed to use the activity inventory as a starting point.

Nicole's Activity Inventory

	Monday	Tuesday	Wednesday	Thursday	Friday	Saturday	Sunday
6–7 A.M.	Sleep	Sleep	Sleep	Sleep	In bed (1)	Sleep	Sleep
7–8 A.M.	Sleep	Sleep	In bed (0)	In bed (1)	In bed (1)	Sleep	Sleep
8–9 A.M.	In bed (2)	Sleep/In bed (1)	In bed (0)	In bed (1)	In bed (0)	In bed (1)	Sleep/In bed (2)
9–10 A.M.	In bed (1)	Breakfast, showered (3)	In bed/games on phone (2–3)	Breakfast and lounging around (2)	In bed (1), breakfast, fed dog (3)	Relaxed in the TV room (2)	In bed (2)
10–11 A.M.	In bed (1) Feed dog (2)	Chat with parents; Drove to Dr's appointment (3–4)	Fed and walked dog (4)	Showered, dressed, fed dog (3)	Walked dog for 20 min (3–4); Sat and stared out the window (1)	Brunch with Keith (4)	In bed (2)
11 A.M.–12 P.M.	Watched TV (2)	Dr. appointment (3)	Picked up groceries (4)	Emptied dishwasher, Cleaned (4)	Watched TV (2)	Shopping with Keith (5)	Internet (2)
12–1 P.M.	TV/Lunch (2)	Lunch (2)	Bite to eat (3)	Lunch (2)	Lunch/TV (2)	Shopping (4–5)	Lunch/TV (2)
1–2 P.M.	Watched TV (2)	Sleep	Listened to music (4)	Nap/In bed (1)	Watched TV (2)	Walked dog (3), TV (2)	Watched TV (2)
2–3 P.M.	Played games on phone (3)	In bed (2)	Nap/In bed (2)	Soak in tub (3)	Sleep	Watched TV (2)	Games on phone, internet (2–3)
3–4 P.M.	Played games on phone (3)	Checked Facebook (2)	Rested on the couch (1–2)	Listened to music (3–4)	In bed (2)	Watched TV, slept (2)	Watched TV (2)

(continued)

Nicole's Activity Inventory *(continued)*

	Monday	Tuesday	Wednesday	Thursday	Friday	Saturday	Sunday
4–5 P.M.	Napping/In bed (2)	Tried to read (3)	Couch (1), helped with supper (3)	Watched TV (3)	Got showered, walked dog (3–4)	Helped prepare supper, listed to music (4)	Prepared to go out (3)
5–6 P.M.	Dinner with Keith (4–5)	Played with dog (3–4)	Dinner with Keith (5)	Walked dog with a friend (6)	Dinner with Keith (4–5)	Dinner with Keith (5)	Dinner at parents' (6)
6–7 P.M.	Watched TV (3)	Dinner alone (2)	Watched TV with Keith (3)	Dinner with Keith (4–5)	Got ready to go out (3–4)	Went for a walk with Keith (5)	Dinner at parents (6)
7–8 P.M.	Watched TV (2)	Chatted with friend (5)/video games (3)	Watched TV with Keith (3)	Played cribbage with Keith (5)	Escape room with Keith and friends (6)	Watched TV (3)	Drove home, watched TV (3)
8–9 P.M.	Watched TV (2)	Video games (3–4)	Watched TV alone (2)	Watched TV (3)	Drove home (4)	Tired, went to bed (2)	Planted some indoor plants (4)
9–10 P.M.	Checked email, responded to texts (4)	Watched TV (2)	Watched TV alone (2)	Watched TV (2)	In bed (2)	In bed (2)	Watched TV (2)
10–11 P.M.	Get ready for bed (2)	In bed (2)	In bed (2)	Scrolling on phone (2)	In bed (1–2)	In bed (2), Sleep	Watched TV (2)
11 P.M.–6 A.M.	Difficulty getting to sleep (0)/Sleep	In bed (2)/Sleep	Sleep	In bed/Sleep	Sleep/Up from 1:30–3:00; difficulty sleeping (0)	Sleep	Watched TV, trouble sleeping, thinking too much (0)

0 = very depressed; 10 = feeling very good

From there, Nicole and Keith worked together to schedule more activities—activities that were enjoyable and activities that were task-focused. And they tried to be systematic about it. Each night, Keith and Nicole would add three things that Nicole could do the next day that were enjoyable and three things that brought her a sense of accomplishment. They started out small, and Keith mentioned that it might take some time before Nicole started to experience pleasure or mastery. "The key is to keep at it," Keith said, "even when you don't feel like it." Eventually, Nicole was able to adjust to this more active schedule and started to reap some of the rewards. Bit by bit, the couple worked on adding more. The key for Nicole was that she didn't feel judged but felt supported to reactivate. She knew that Keith was "pushing" this because he loved her. And the couple was able to talk openly about how to balance some pushing without pushing too much.

5. Come Up with a Plan

If you and your partner were able to work through and review an activity inventory, great. I hope you were able to see some patterns that you could change bit by bit. The next step is to come up with a plan. If your partner wasn't able to complete an activity inventory or you weren't able to review it together, I hope you won't be too discouraged. Coming up with a plan will still be helpful; you just may not have the benefit of knowing what specific activities help boost your partner's mood and those that drag them down. However, through the power of observation, I am sure you can come up with some ideas.

The goal in making a plan is to help your partner gain momentum. It is so easy to backslide if your partner is feeling really down or off. With your partner's agreement, you will want to try to schedule some activities for each day. Some activities should focus on pleasure, and some should focus on accomplishments. There is no rule for this, but generally starting with about three of each is helpful.

There are a couple of reasons pleasure is so important. First, we know that people tend to feel less depressed when they have experiences they enjoy. Of course, it's a bit of a double-edged sword because depression can numb the experiences of pleasure. Even if there is no enjoyment, however, it would still be helpful for your partner to do enjoyable things. By continuing to persevere, your partner will slowly start to experience pleasure again. The other reason it is important to do pleasurable things has to do with how people think about themselves when depressed. They often have a ton of negative thoughts about themselves, those around them, and their future. Doing pleasurable things sends different messages to your partner . . . messages that they are worth caring for, that they have a right to experience joy, that they do deserve happiness. They may not believe it at first, but acting from the outside in (instead of the inside out)—from a plan instead of feelings—will help to change how your partner is behaving, feeling, and thinking.

To come up with pleasurable activities, you can use the list provided in the box on pages 72–73. Ask yourself what your partner once found rewarding but no longer thinks they will enjoy or currently engages in less often. Are there things they have never tried that might fit with who they are?

Try to determine what could be increased and decreased. Ultimately, you want to increase things that involve approach behavior, activity, and connectedness and reduce things that are sedentary, avoidant, or passive. Here are some ideas:

- If you and your partner completed the activity inventory, you could start there. What activities on the inventory helped your partner feel better?
- Could they continue trying to do these activities? (Choose a few that they would like to continue doing.)
- Are there activities that your partner can include in their new routine?
- Are there things your partner could do to help them through the parts of the day that are the worst for them?
- What are some activities that your partner used to enjoy but is no longer doing? Could the two of you experiment with trying some of these?
- What are your partner's values? What kind of relationships do they want to have with family or friends? What kind of partner do they want to be? What kind of parent would they want to be? How do they want to grow as a person? Sometimes listing your values can be a good starting point. It can help you find activities that are consistent with those values and that increase motivation and incentive to work on.
- What gives your partner meaning? Could they choose some activities that would help them feel more accomplishment?
- Make sure that the pleasure and accomplishment activities are doable. It's better for your partner to start small and build up than to start too big and feel like giving up.

- Try to increase physical activity. This will help improve your partner's mood as well.

- What is your partner avoiding? How are they avoiding? Are they sleeping in too much, napping too often, drinking too frequently, numbing out on their phone? Some distractions can be helpful in the short term, but trying to minimize these will help in the long run.

- Plan for activities that involve social connection. Maybe your partner could reach out to people they haven't seen in a long time. Perhaps they could join a group or volunteer in an organization to meet new people.

With all these activities, it's important to make sure you and your partner are on the same page. Take time to set up the ground rules. This way you'll know when you're pushing too much or not enough. Try to schedule activities that follow a plan, not a mood.

Depending on the severity of your partner's depression, they may benefit more from seeing a qualified mental health professional who practices behavioral activation or cognitive-behavioral therapy. In this case, you might be able to help your partner do some of the "homework" that has been assigned in therapy. If your partner isn't yet willing to see someone for therapy, working on some of these strategies might still help shift their mood, and they may come around to see the benefit of working with a professional.

If your partner's depression is not too incapacitating, working through some of these strategies with them will likely be helpful. If you want more information on how to do behavioral activation, check out *The Behavioral Activation Workbook for Depression* by Drs. Stephen R. Swallow and Nina Josefowitz.

Keep at it. Helping your partner become more active is likely to be beneficial.

6

Helping Your Partner Change Negative Thinking

Janani and Ganesh had been married for two years. Janani struggled with depression, and Ganesh tried his best to be supportive. One Sunday morning, Janani was sitting on the couch, lost in her thoughts and looking despondent. Ganesh brewed Janani a coffee and put it down beside her with an issue of *Homes and Gardens.* "I thought you might like to read this," Ganesh said. "You liked planning out our garden for the season last year and the year before."

Janani glanced down at the magazine and was flooded with negative thoughts. *Ganesh must think that all I do is sit here and dwell on my thoughts. He thinks I'm too lazy to do anything. He's right. I'm pathetic.* Janani pushed the magazine aside and looked tearful. Ganesh was surprised by Janani's reaction. He thought this would lift her mood a bit and help her focus on the warm months ahead. "What's wrong?" Ganesh asked. "I thought you would like this." Janani felt helpless, and her negative thinking quickly spiraled into self-doubt and despair: *I'll never be able to pull myself out of this. I'm such a burden.*

You can probably recall similar scenarios. You try to do something to lift your partner's mood and it falls flat or makes the situation worse. How could such a benign and loving gesture be received so differently than intended?

To understand how this can happen, try to envision what it would be like to put on a pair of glasses that were tinted with hues of self-hatred. Glasses that could allow you to see only the worst in yourself, masterfully tracking every failure and incapable of recalling successes. Lenses that saw only the negative and deflected the positives. Glasses that amplified your view of how worthless, unlovable, despicable, or incompetent you are. This is the lens of depression.

It's hard to understand, and it's painful to witness, but when your partner is depressed, their view of themself, others, and their future is dark and bleak.

Your partner isn't trying to be negative. Sadly, this is the typical experience of depression. When people are depressed, every aspect of their thinking becomes negatively skewed. What they pay attention to becomes biased. It's as though they were wearing blinders, seeing only the negative. They remember negative things and don't seem able to recall good, happy, or even neutral events. They tend to interpret neutral events in a negative light and dismiss or think positive situations are the exception and not the rule.

Negative Automatic Thoughts

Depression fills the mind with negative automatic thoughts. Automatic thoughts are the frequent thoughts that pop into our minds and are not necessarily rational or based on reality. Every day, each of us experiences hundreds of automatic thoughts. You've likely already experienced several automatic thoughts while reading this book: *I hope this book will be useful. I hope this chapter will be interesting. Will I be able to understand all of this? More importantly, will I be able to implement these strategies with my partner?* When people are not depressed, there is a higher ratio of positive to negative thoughts. With depression, however, negative thoughts tend to consume the mind. Over time, negative thinking can become the default way of thinking.

Do you remember when you first learned to drive a car? At the beginning, you were acutely aware of how much pressure was placed on the gas or brakes. You were sure to keep your hands in the ten and two o'clock positions of the steering wheel. You were hypervigilant to everything that was happening outside of the windshield. Every skill took a conscious and deliberate effort. You wouldn't dare have the radio on—it would be too distracting for you as a young, frightened driver. But after a month or two, you were comfortable, driving with a coffee in your hand, listening to music, chatting with friends, and enjoying the landscape outside of your window. How did all of that happen? Over time, as you become more adept at driving, these skills become automatic. They start to be second nature for you. You no longer need to think about it, because your brain has figured out a way to automate these skills.

Much like driving a car, the nature of depression means that negative thinking becomes the default way of thinking. It's the first response, and the more negative thoughts come up, the more the pattern of negative thinking takes hold. Your partner's negative thinking has, over time, become automatic. The problem with negative thinking being the default mode is that your partner never questions whether a particular thought is true. They don't stop and ask, "Wait a second. Is this even true? Is this thought I have about myself valid?" Without questioning and checking out the truth in their beliefs, your partner's negative thoughts eventually become ingrained and increasingly difficult to change.

Identifying Negative Thinking Patterns

In Chapter 1 you learned that negative thinking is part of the experience of depression. In Chapter 3 you were introduced to how CBT can help people challenge negative thoughts to see that they are either not true or not helpful or both. You can contribute to this effort by gently helping your partner recognize how their negative thought patterns may be contributing to their depression. The first step is to become familiar with the thinking traps that are likely to snare your partner. Take a moment to review the table on pages 85–86.

How to Tackle Thinking Traps with Your Partner

Now that you're familiar with some of the thinking traps, try to be on the lookout for which ones are most relevant to your partner. Do they tend to personalize, catastrophize, or disqualify the positives?

Trying to engage your partner in tackling thinking traps can be challenging. Start by picking a time when you're both calm. If your partner is agreeable, try to come up with a plan for how you can both start to identify and tackle these thinking traps. Rather than being critical or judgmental, the goal is to help your partner see things differently. You need to be on the same page for this to be successful.

You might want to briefly explain how negative thinking impacts depression and describe some of the thinking traps listed in the thinking errors table. You could ask your partner if they think that any of these apply to them.

Take time to explore your partner's thoughts as they come up in different situations or when they are feeling distressed or overwhelmed. It could be a small disagreement, a mistake that was made, or a time when they chastised themself for staying in bed too long.

To keep track of these thinking traps, it's helpful to write down what happened, what your partner was specifically thinking, and what emotion they

Typical Thinking Errors in Depression

Thinking traps	Definition	Example
Catastrophizing	Making negative predictions about the future.	Tim is waiting for the results of a medical test. Even though the doctor's office could be calling for a routine follow-up or to discuss something minor, Tim's mind races to the most terrifying possibilities: *What if I have cancer? I will be incapacitated and unable to work*. Tim ignores the fact that there may be other more likely (and less serious) explanations.
All-or-nothing thinking	Seeing things as "black or white," without seeing the gray. Viewing things as either all good or all bad, with no in between.	Chris notices a mistake on one of his PowerPoint slides. *The whole presentation is ruined. I'm a failure.*
Labeling	Assigning a global, negative label to yourself (or others) based on a single event or characteristic.	John forgets to return a phone call and thinks, *I'm a failure. I can't do anything right. I'm worthless.*
Should statements	Holding rigid, unrealistic, or overly critical expectations of oneself; thinking that people or things must be a certain way.	Tina is looking at her to-do list and thinking, *I should be more productive. I should be able to handle things better. I should be able to figure this out.*
Mind reading	Assuming that others are thinking negatively about you.	Sarina is having dinner with her partner, Michael, who isn't very talkative. Sarina assumes that Michael is unhappy with her.
Emotional reasoning	Believing something is true because it "feels" that way.	Elizabeth is well prepared for her presentation but is feeling nervous. *I feel anxious right now. That must mean I'm going to screw this up. If I feel this nervous, I must not be ready. Everyone will think I'm incompetent.*

(continued)

Typical Thinking Errors in Depression *(continued)*

Thinking traps	Definition	Example
Mental filter	Focusing solely on the negative aspects of a situation while ignoring any positive one.	Katerina's boss made many positive comments on a report she submitted. He also pointed out one minor correction. Although Katerina impressed her boss, she could only think about that one comment and kept beating herself up for the mistake. She felt like a failure.
Overgeneralization	Taking one negative event or experience and applying it across the board, making broad, sweeping conclusions based on limited evidence.	Lisa had a small disagreement with a friend. She later reflected, *That conversation went poorly. No one will ever want to be my friend. I always mess things up in relationships.*
Personalization	Believing you are responsible for negative things, even though you're not.	Tom's partner was in a bad mood. Tom assumes that he must have done something wrong.
Minimizing or disqualifying the positive	Dismissing positive experiences, achievements, or compliments as irrelevant.	Pascale gets positive feedback on an assignment and thinks, *They're just saying that to be nice. It was luck. It doesn't mean anything; I'm still not good enough.*

felt at the time (sad, frustrated, angry, anxious). Once you have a sense of your partner's thoughts, see if you can both identify the thinking trap that is most relevant. For example, if your partner thought, *I didn't call [friend's name]. They are never going to speak to me again,* this would be an example of catastrophizing. If they thought, *I'm always screwing up. I'll never succeed,* this would be overgeneralization.

Once you and your partner have identified some of these thoughts, you can critically evaluate them. It's important to be patient and come up with a strategy that is palatable for both of you. Does your partner want your input? How will you know when it's enough but not too much? Some open discussion about the ground rules might be prudent.

TRY THIS: USE A COLOR-CODING SCHEME TO GAUGE YOUR PARTNER'S WILLINGNESS

If it's easier, you could even come up with a coding scheme that you both agree on that indicates how your partner is handling this exercise. For instance, you could have a color code of green, yellow, and red. Green means "I am open to reviewing my thoughts. You have a green light." Yellow means "Proceed with caution. I am feeling vulnerable right now. I want to do this, but I don't want to be pushed too much." Red means "Let's cut our losses and stop doing this for now. I don't want to say something I'll regret."

When your partner is ready and willing to review their thoughts, start out by checking the evidence. *You want to think about it as though you are putting the thoughts on trial.* What gets admitted as evidence are facts, not feelings or interpretations of facts.

- What evidence supports this thought?
- What evidence contradicts this thought?
- Is there another way to look at this situation? Are there alternative explanations?
- What would you say to a friend if they were thinking this way? (Or what would a friend say to me if they knew I had this thought?)
- Is there another way of thinking about the situation that is more balanced, realistic, or helpful?

Looking at the evidence is easier said than done. It may take some time, but people tend to improve using this exercise because they become more aware of those sneaky negative thoughts. If you want an excellent book that will help your partner learn more about changing their thinking, I recommend *Mind over Mood* by Greenberger and Padesky.

Let's assume that a situation occurred last week. You made plans for the two of you to meet up with some friends for dinner. Your partner canceled at the last minute, claiming that they were feeling too tired and overwhelmed. At the time, you were disappointed and frustrated, but that's water under the bridge and you are now trying to help your partner deal with their negative thoughts. "You seemed really upset last week when we needed to cancel our plans." "Yeah," your partner admits, "I felt really sad and hopeless." "What were you thinking?" you ask. "That I'm always letting people down," your partner expresses. You write this thought down.

What thinking trap is this an example of?" Together, you might want to look at the list in the Typical Thinking Errors in Depression table. In this case, you would conclude that this was overgeneralizing. The next step is to help your partner examine the evidence. You might start by validating your partner's experience: "I understand that you're feeling down right now, and the thought that you are always letting people down must feel really heavy. Can we look at this thought together? What is the evidence that you are *always* letting people down?" "Well," your partner states, "it sucks that we missed going out for dinner." "True, that was disappointing," you reply. "Is there other evidence that you always let others down?"

You want to allow your partner to come up with some other examples that support their thought and validate these. This is important so you don't jump too quickly to looking for evidence that refutes the thought—doing so only makes the evaluation of your partner's thought seem one-sided and biased. By examining *both* sides of the equation (evidence that supports the belief and evidence that contradicts the belief), your partner will be able to sift through the information and come up with alternative thoughts that are more balanced and that incorporate all the evidence. They will be able to see themself with clear glasses.

Once you have reviewed some of the evidence that supports their thought, it's time to switch gears and look at the evidence that is not consistent with the thought. For example,

- Can you think of times when you did something that others appreciated?
- Can you recall times when you said or did something that made others happy?
- What do your friends or family say? Do they always view you as letting them down?

You could say, "I know you're disappointed, but one cancellation doesn't mean that you always let people down. Everyone has tough days and needs to take care of themselves sometimes." (Be prepared to get some yes-butting as it may take time for your partner to see things more objectively. A good dose of patience will help here.)

Encourage your partner to think about recent examples, even small ones, when they were reliable or supported someone. You might think of an example or two yourself. For example, "Yesterday, you helped me make dinner. I appreciated that," or "Your friend thanked you for taking the time to listen to them when they were feeling bummed out." The idea is to help your partner see that the initial thought—in this case, *I'm always letting people down*—is too broad or exaggerated.

Next, you want to help your partner reframe the thought by coming up with alternatives that are more balanced and consider both sides of the evidence. For example, "Although it was disappointing to cancel on dinner last week, I don't always let people down. In fact, there are lots of times when I have been there for others and supported them. Canceling on dinner doesn't mean that I am *always* letting people down." Developing balanced thoughts that integrate the evidence that both supports the thought and doesn't support the thought will make the new thoughts more believable to your partner and more likely to sink in. The goal is to be evidence-based in our thinking—not overly positive, but evidence-based. It's not the power of positive thinking but the power of non-negative or realistic thinking that will help to reduce depression.

When working through different thinking traps, your partner might at times come up with a bunch of thoughts all at once. To take the previous canceled dinner example, they might have claimed, "I'm such a disappointment [labeling]. I'm always letting people down [overgeneralizing]. My friends probably don't want to be around me anymore [mind-reading]. I'm just a burden to everyone [mind-reading, catastrophizing]. I can't do anything right [all-or-nothing thinking]." When there are multiple thoughts at once, it's important to tackle one at a time. Write each of them down and pick one to start with.

It isn't necessary to provide a label to these thinking traps; however, it can sometimes be helpful to do so. Similar thinking traps tend to come up repeatedly. By recognizing and understanding some of the main thinking traps your partner gets into, you can help identify them as they arise. You could even be a bit playful with the process. For example, when your partner makes a comment like "I should be more productive; I should push harder" you might help identify *should* statements by saying "Stop *should*ing on yourself, honey." If your partner accidentally burns dinner and says, "Ugh, the whole evening is ruined," you could remind them not to fall for the all-or-nothing thinking trap. Before you do this, it might be smart to check with your partner to see if some gentle reminders would be helpful to them.

Using Behavioral Activation to Help Change Thinking

In Chapter 5, we reviewed some strategies for helping your partner become more activated. Hopefully you were able to come up with a systematic schedule that helped them feel better by avoiding less and engaging in more activities that provided a sense of pleasure and feeling of accomplishment. Behavioral activation can also be used to tackle negative thinking. Remember the recommendation to start with three pleasure and three accomplishment activities? You can also help your partner by spending time reviewing how these activities went. What did they learn from doing this? Are there activities that helped them feel better? If so, what were they thinking about themself when this happened? You might want to point out that they seemed more confident when they went to the store with you or accomplished some task. Did they feel more confident? What thoughts did they have? How about when they pushed themself to visit a friend. How did that go? Did they enjoy it? Did they laugh more than they thought they would? What can they conclude from this?

When we change our behavior in positive ways, we also change our thinking. And starting to think differently, in turn, improves our behavior. By feeling more confident and capable, your partner will start to engage more. And by engaging more, your partner will feel more confident and capable.

When doing behavioral activation, there are also times when you can check on what your partner is thinking about the activity and use this information to challenge their beliefs. For example, let's assume that your partner was invited out to a friend's place for lunch. You could ask them, on a scale from 0 to 10 (with zero being no enjoyment and 10 being the most enjoyment they've ever had), how much pleasure they predict they will have. If they anticipate a 2/10 in enjoyment, then it makes sense they don't want to go. If that was your prediction, you would probably stay at home in your pajamas too. But what if you tested this prediction (remember, action precedes motivation—act first and the motivation will likely follow)? Your partner goes and it turns out to be a 5/10 or 6/10 instead of a 2/10. It wasn't groundbreaking, but it went better than expected. What can they learn from that? They may have learned that, because of their depression, they are underestimating the value of being active and engaging with others. If that is the case, maybe the next time they have a similar prediction they could remember what happened; that their predictions may not be very accurate and how they feel is not a good predictor of the outcome.

Using a Thought Record to Capture and Change Thinking

With some practice, your partner will understand how thoughts impact feelings and behavior. They will also be able to more regularly catch negative automatic thoughts as they occur and learn to change them so that they are more adaptive and helpful, which will help improve their mood.

The thought record is another useful tool for catching and changing negative thinking. The basic idea is to have your partner record their thoughts as they occur in the moment. Because we all have hundreds of automatic thoughts each day, your partner isn't going to record all of them, just the ones that are related to a noticeable shift in their mood. When you (or they) observe a shift in their mood, like an increase in sadness or a jump in anxiety, write it down and figure out what thoughts contributed to their mood.

Start by writing down what happened or what was going on when your partner's mood changed. Then ask, "What were you thinking just before you started to feel that way?" Write down the automatic thoughts. Next, write down what your partner's mood was and how intense it felt from zero (*not intense at all*) to 100 (*the most intense I have ever experienced*). Following this, you can work through different steps with your partner. For instance, you may want to work together to determine what thinking traps they fell into.

The next step is to discuss the evidence that supports the thought and the evidence that doesn't support the thought. Take your time with this and try to flesh this out. You really want to put these thoughts on trial. It is often helpful to think of a thought as a hypothesis rather than a fact. In other words, just because your partner has a particular thought doesn't mean that it's necessarily true. There could be other explanations that are more accurate or helpful.

After reviewing the evidence, see if you and your partner can come up with a more balanced and helpful thought. The last step involves rating your partner's mood again to see if it changed (see the table on page 92 for an example).

If your partner's mood changed, great! Coming up with a more balanced thought was likely helpful. Keep at it. If it didn't change or didn't shift that much, you may have to troubleshoot a bit:

Example of a Thought Record	
Situation	My partner seemed distracted during a conversation we had. They didn't respond right away and didn't ask how I was feeling.
Automatic thought	"They don't care about me. I'm not important to them. They're probably tired of me."
Mood rating (0–100)	Sadness (80)
Step 1: What were the thinking traps?	Mind Reading: "They don't care about me." Labeling: "I'm not important to them." Catastrophizing: "They're probably tired of me."
Step 2: Evidence for the thought	My partner seemed distracted during the conversation. They didn't ask how I was feeling at that moment.
Step 3: Evidence against the thought	My partner has been a huge support to me. They often ask how I'm doing. They've helped me through many tough times. They've expressed care for me in other ways. They've been stressed at work lately, which could explain why they were distracted. They often tell me they love me. They often show their love and affection in small ways throughout the day.
Step 4: Balanced thought	"Just because my partner seemed distracted today, that doesn't mean they don't care. They've shown me tons of love and support. Maybe they were dealing with their own stress and didn't notice how I was feeling. It's possible that I misread the situation."
Step 5: Rerate mood (0–100)	40

- One possibility is that the thoughts your partner identified weren't the ones that were really impacting their emotions. In this case, try to zero in on the thoughts that were driving the emotion.
- Another possibility is that the evidence wasn't evaluated fully enough.
- A third possibility is that the balanced thought they came up with wasn't believable or didn't incorporate all the evidence.

Be patient with this. Changing automatic thoughts takes practice, and it's going to take some time and effort to get good at it. Be persistent—it can really help your partner to change their thinking and, in turn, help them feel better.

Although you don't need to use a thought record, there is something about writing thoughts down that is helpful. It allows your partner to focus on one thought at a time instead of having a stream of thoughts cascade through their mind. Writing it down can also help them evaluate the thought more systematically. With time and practice, they will be able to catch and change thoughts in the moment. If your partner would prefer to complete thought records on their phone, there are several apps that are based on cognitive-behavioral principles that your partner can download on their phone or tablet: MoodTools, CBT Thought Diary, Sanvello, and Moodfit are some examples.

Troubleshooting

Your partner may not be willing to talk about their thinking traps or work through a thought record with you. If that's the case, try not to take it personally. It's a tall task, and maybe now isn't the time. You may also find that your partner gets frustrated by the suggestion that they should monitor their thoughts or try to change them ("You don't understand what I am going through or how hard this is"). If that happens, this is your cue to back off for now and try to revisit another time. Give your partner some space and try to support them in other ways (remember, connect first—see Chapter 2). Later, you might be able to help them see things more objectively by pointing out alternative perspectives to the thoughts they express in your day-to-day interactions. They might eventually come around and see the benefits of systematically working through their automatic thoughts.

Here are some things to consider:

1. ***Get their consent:*** Helping to change your partner's thoughts requires that they are a willing participant. Although you can help your partner see alternative perspectives, you won't make much (if any) progress if they are resistant or unmotivated to do this.

2. ***Be patient and understanding:*** Changing negative thinking takes a lot of time and effort. This isn't going to happen overnight. Some days you might feel as though you are only planting a seed, whereas other days you might see some real progress. Take it one step at a time.

3. ***Communicate openly:*** Be honest about what you are both going through and try to create a supportive environment for each other. They will need to feel comfortable sharing their thoughts without judgment for this to be helpful.

4. ***Join them:*** The truth is that we all have thoughts that are biased or that we could work on changing. You might consider doing a thought record for yourself and sharing your experiences with your partner. This can help your partner feel less alone and more willing to try.

5. ***Be consistent:*** The key to success in changing thinking is to regularly practice these strategies. Your partner's thoughts will take time to change. They have been thinking this way for a long time. Be patient. You'll get there eventually.

Finally, if your partner is struggling with persistent negative thinking, it may be more fruitful for them to see a psychologist or other health professional. A therapist who practices evidence-based treatments like cognitive-behavioral therapy can provide expertise and support in identifying and challenging negative thoughts.

Negative automatic thoughts are also typically related to deeper underlying beliefs like "I am worthless," "I'm incompetent," or "I'm unlovable." A well-trained expert can best help your partner identify and modify some of these deeper beliefs that may be contributing to your partner's negative automatic thoughts.

Regardless of whether you or a professional is the one to help, when your partner's negative thinking begins to change, they will better manage their emotions, develop healthier coping strategies, communicate more effectively with you, and feel better. Your relationship will also strengthen. You will also feel better about your partner, your relationship, and yourself. It's a lot of work, but it's worth the effort to get negative thinking on track.

7

Being Aware of Warning Signs and Managing Expectations

My hope is that you've experienced some breakthroughs and successes as you've worked through the preceding chapters. Perhaps your partner was open to the idea of getting professional help for depression and is now benefiting from psychotherapy or medication. Maybe your efforts to connect first have helped your partner feel validated and supported and provided you with some momentum to work on other strategies. Behavioral activation may have helped your partner get unstuck, even if just a little. The hard work to help your partner change negative thinking may have begun to pay off.

If you've experienced some success—even small gains—great, keep at it. The hard part now is being deliberate and systematic about continuous improvement. But if your experience so far is not exactly what you would define as "success," you might feel you've tried everything and nothing seems to work. Don't give up. Change is super difficult and takes time. Take another stab at some of the strategies described in Chapters 4–6. Is it possible to approach these differently? You might consider discussing other treatment options with your partner. Alternatively, you may need to step back for a bit and catch your breath before you feel ready to try again.

This chapter focuses on some warning signs to be aware of and strategies for managing them as you move forward. Understanding indicators that your partner's depression is returning, not improving, or getting worse, or they are at risk of harming themself, and knowing what to do, can help you best support your partner and navigate these emotional complexities.

Remember, Depression Is Episodic and Recurrent

Depression comes and goes. For some people, episodes of depression are short, whereas for others they can last for months or longer. Approximately 40% of individuals with major depressive disorder will recover within three months, and about 80% typically recover within a year. However, some people experience depression that continues for long periods of time. Bipolar disorder is typically a lifelong problem, although the episodes of mania/hypomania or depression may come and go.

Your partner may start to feel better, and their depression might improve, only to return at some point later. Most individuals with depression (50–90%) experience multiple subsequent episodes. The odds of experiencing another episode also tend to increase each time someone experiences depression. For example, the probability of experiencing future depression after an initial episode is about 50%. If your partner experiences two episodes, the chances of future depression are higher—about 70%. The odds increase to about 90% after three episodes.

Depression affects people differently. Some people may experience only a few episodes in their lifetime, whereas others might have ongoing challenges. Your partner's prognosis can significantly improve by getting the right treatment. For example, CBT can effectively treat depression and reduce the risk that it will return (see Chapter 3).

Preparing yourself for the possibility of relapse can be helpful. Be on the lookout for signs that your partner's depression may be returning (see Chapter 1):

- A shift back toward sadness or irritability
- Loss of interest in things that used to give your partner a sense of purpose or pleasure
- Failure of the usual coping mechanisms, leaving your partner feeling either overwhelmed or indifferent
- A new sense of worthlessness or guilt over things they have done or not done
- Increased isolation and pulling away from you or others
- Reappearance of old patterns of negative thinking

You will likely have to help your partner through different dark periods, but seeing depression as an episodic problem can help you recognize that it is not usually permanent. In addition, by working through the strategies outlined in this book, you've developed some skills to help when your partner is experiencing another episode and can provide hope that things will improve again.

During the times your partner is doing well, continue working on ways to maintain their mental health and minimize relapse. For example, you can help your partner stay engaged with their treatment, whether that is therapy, medication, or other strategies. Even when your partner is feeling better, encourage them to continue doing what works—behavioral activation and keeping their thinking in check. Implementing these strategies can reduce the risk that depression will return. If it does, you will be prepared by keeping an eye out for early warning signs of relapse. By catching this early, you can help your partner before things get worse.

What If My Partner's Depression Is Not Improving?

Sometimes depression is more chronic, severe, and unremitting. Your partner may have tried several types of antidepressant medication or different therapies with no mood improvements. You might both feel stuck and hopeless. It's incredibly disheartening and frustrating when nothing you've tried seems to work. Don't give up hope. Just as there are many ways people can become depressed, there are many ways out of depression.

After you land on your feet following this distressing and disappointing outcome, see if your partner is willing to meet with their health care provider to explore new options. For example, are there other medications that might be worth a shot? Would it be helpful to try another form of therapy that your partner hasn't yet attempted? Perhaps a particular therapy provider wasn't all that helpful. Would working with someone else be the solution?

When depression is more severe and chronic, other medical alternatives are available as well, such as transcranial magnetic stimulation, electroconvulsive therapy (discussed in Chapter 3), or ketamine (an anesthetic shown to provide fast-acting relief for individuals with depression who haven't responded well to other treatments). No treatment is without risks, so have your partner contact their family doctor or psychiatrist to weigh the pros and cons of interventional psychiatry options.

One of the toughest parts of supporting someone with treatment-resistant depression is that progress can feel painfully slow. While you and your partner are exploring other treatment options, try to have them keep up with some behavioral activation and basic lifestyle routines. Encourage your partner to stick to a routine—like getting up at the same time, showering, and eating regularly—even small steps can make a difference. With a good dose of support, you may even gently try to help your partner see things less negatively. These aren't replacements for psychological or medical treatments, but they can help. One step at a time. The victories may be small during this period (like your partner getting out of bed, showering, or agreeing to do something enjoyable), but try to celebrate them even if they seem trivial. Encouragement and gentle prompting might help your partner follow a routine and begin to do more activities that will help them feel better.

What if nothing works? This can feel exhausting and overwhelming for both of you. Depression can be stubborn, and watching your partner struggle day after day without relief takes an emotional toll on you too. Make sure to take care of yourself as well. Your well-being is also important, and keeping yourself in the equation is essential. You won't be a help to your partner or yourself if you burn out. Try to maximize your own mental and physical well-being as much as you can. Keep up your strength by seeking support for yourself, ensuring you get enough rest, or acknowledging when you need time away. The second part of this book, beginning with the next chapter, focuses on supporting yourself through your partner's depression.

Understanding Suicide Risk

Millions of individuals struggle with suicidal thoughts, and more than 700,000 people die by suicide each year. Suicide is the tenth-leading cause of death globally and the ninth-leading cause in North America.

If your partner is experiencing suicidal thoughts, you are probably in constant fear that they may harm themself or end their life. Coping with the possibility that your partner may take their life can be overwhelming. Although you might feel tremendous pressure to "save" them, you also feel paralyzed, unsure what to say or do. These fears are common and valid. The fear of losing a loved one to suicide is a deeply distressing reality for many, especially if the partner is struggling with severe depression or has previously expressed or acted on suicidal thoughts.

There are many risk factors for suicide. For instance, suicide is associated with various mental health problems, such as depression. Impulsivity, physical and sexual abuse, a history of trauma, chronic pain, alcohol and substance abuse, a family history of suicide, relationship or job loss, lack of social support, feeling like a burden, aggressive tendencies, major physical illness, and past attempts are all correlated with risk for suicide.

However, just because an *association* exists doesn't mean that this is the *cause.* It only means that there is a relationship between the two variables. If I told you that there is a strong relationship between the number of churches, synagogues, mosques, or temples in a city and the number of nightclubs, you might think that there is a link between being religious and partying. However, there could be another, more viable, explanation for this relationship. In this instance, the other explanation could be the population of the city—as the number of people increase, the number of religious buildings and nightclubs independently increase to accommodate the population growth. Similarly, just the fact that depression and suicide are associated doesn't mean that depression causes suicide. Depression is a risk factor for suicide, but many people with depression don't have suicidal thoughts and many individuals who experience suicidal thoughts don't act on them.

So, what does increase the odds that someone with suicidal thoughts will act on them? Four factors seem to play a critical role: pain, hopelessness, lack of connection, and capability.

Pain

Feeling burdened with pain increases the likelihood of suicidal thoughts. This pain can be psychological or physical and may stem from several things, including symptoms of depression, relationship breakups, job loss, or medical conditions. When people feel their life is painful or miserable, they are naturally inclined to try to avoid or escape pain. They are more likely to think about finding a way out. Your partner may feel they have been struggling with their depression or bipolar disorder for far too long and are increasingly a burden on you and others. These mental health conditions can cloud judgment, making it difficult for your partner to see a way out of their emotional suffering. If they have been wrestling with chronic pain, they may understandably want to find a way out. They may feel trapped in a cycle of despair and perceive suicide as the only way to escape the pain they're experiencing. In these moments the emotional distress can outweigh any thoughts of potential relief, leading to a sense of finality.

Hopelessness

The experience of pain is not enough to increase the desire for suicide. When pain is combined with hopelessness, however, suicidal urges emerge. For example, if your partner is in severe psychological pain but believes that they might get through this with your help or the assistance of a mental health professional, they will likely work on trying to improve their circumstances and push for a brighter future. If, on the other hand, they are completely hopeless and believe that their depression (or other psychological or physical pain) won't improve, they may start to think about suicide as a possible way out.

Connectedness

Pain and hopelessness push someone away from a desire to live, whereas connectedness pulls them toward a desire to live. Connectedness includes how close your partner feels in their relationships with you, family, and close friends. It also has to do with having meaning and purpose in life and a valued role or identity in their world. Feeling connected and believing that something or someone important beyond self is there can make life worth living. Suicidal urges intensify when the pain your partner experiences is greater than the connectedness they feel.

Capability

Although you want to be sure to monitor your partner and check in with them regularly when they are experiencing suicidal thoughts, the good news is that most people with suicidal thoughts don't attempt suicide. What seems to shift a person from having strong suicidal urges to making attempts is their capability. For example, your partner's capacity for suicide may increase if they have access to things that are lethal (like having a gun in the home) or acquire knowledge of lethal strategies (such as learning online how to end one's life).

Reducing Suicide Risk

The truth is that it is impossible to predict with 100% accuracy whether your partner's suicidal thinking will lead to suicidal behavior. Suicidologist Dr. E. David Klonsky described it as akin to predicting catastrophic weather events. Meteorologists have expertise and knowledge about tornadoes and issue extreme weather alerts on your phone or television when they are about to occur. However, they can't predict days, weeks, or months in advance when such conditions will exist. Uncertainties about your partner, no doubt, increase your own fears and anxieties.

The best you can do is understand the conditions that are most likely to lead to death by suicide. Although you can offer support and try to guide your partner to the right help, you can't fix them. As much as it feels as though this burden falls entirely on your shoulders, you aren't responsible for your partner's actions, nor are you able to predict what they will do.

What you can do is help your partner reduce the risk that suicidal thoughts and actions will occur by helping them decrease pain, increase hope, improve connectedness, and reduce their capability for suicide.

Decrease Pain

As we discussed earlier in the book, you might want to start by acknowledging and validating your partner's emotional pain without dismissing it: "I know you're really hurting, and I'm here for you." Don't avoid talking about suicide. Many people assume that talking about suicide increases the chances that suicide will occur. This is simply not true. Engaging in open, compassionate, and nonjudgmental conversations about suicidal thoughts can reduce risk and serve as a protective factor. Having an open discussion with your partner sends a message that you understand their pain and makes them feel heard and validated. Because your partner may start to recognize that they can talk about what they are going through without fear of judgment, they may be more open to accessing the help they need—help that they might have otherwise avoided.

If they are open to it, help your partner recognize the benefits of seeking professional help, particularly approaches that are supported by scientific evidence (see Chapter 3). Another way to reduce your partner's pain is to promote some of the strategies to engage in behavioral activation and change thinking (see Chapters 5 and 6).

Increase Hope

Gently remind your loved one that, although things seem overwhelming, many strategies and treatments can help them feel better. Encourage them that they will climb out of their depression and that these feelings of hopelessness are temporary. If they have experienced depression previously, see if they can recall how they managed to get out of that episode and reinforce the fact that they are resilient and able to do it again. Help your partner understand that there are effective approaches that can not only help to treat depression but also prevent it from coming back again.

Promote Connection

Help your partner stay connected with you and others. If they've been avoiding and withdrawing from others, help them gradually reconnect in ways that don't pressure them. You might want to make specific plans to reconnect with people. Helping them check out the evidence for some of the thoughts they have about doing this can also be beneficial. For example, your partner may have the thought, "I haven't connected for so long; it's too late. I am embarrassed, and they probably don't want to hear from me." You could help them think differently by examining the evidence. For instance, "If your friend was out of touch for a period because *they* had depression, how would *you* respond if they reached out? Would you shut them out?"

Check in with your partner regularly and do your best to spend quality time together, even if they are tough to be around. Express love, appreciation, and gratitude for who they are and what they have contributed to your life and your relationship. Even though the relationship may be strained now, this will not last forever, and you will be able to strengthen your relationship over time. Help them reconnect with things that used to give them a sense of value and purpose. Fostering connection is vital. Remind your partner how important they are to you—how their family and friends need them in their lives. Try your best to listen actively and offer empathy, support, and validation. Let your partner know that you are invested in them and their well-being.

Create a Safe Environment

Do a walk-through of your place and remove dangerous objects or substances (medications, firearms, sharp objects, ropes). The idea is to create a barrier between your partner and the methods they might use to harm themself or end their life. For instance, you could consider removing alcohol or substances from the home if drinking alcohol or using drugs makes their suicidal behavior more likely. Old medications could be taken to a pharmacist for disposal so that they aren't lying around the house.

Help your partner understand that seeking help is not a sign of weakness but a sign of strength. By being open about needing support, they reduce the desire to resort to harmful coping strategies.

When in a moment of crisis, help your partner focus on immediate, safe distractions that can pull them away from their suicidal thoughts. This could include deep breathing, taking a walk, or watching a favorite show. Help your partner cultivate a sense of self-compassion and work to challenge the harsh inner critic. Finally, try to get your partner to think about their future and to make even small plans.

If you think your partner is in imminent danger, it's critical to seek professional help, like calling a therapist or a suicide prevention hotline, or even dialing 911.

Developing a Safety Plan

Creating a plan collaboratively with your partner can ensure their safety and reduce the risk of suicide. The main idea is to construct a set of coping strategies and sources of support ahead of time that can be used when there is a crisis or suicidal thinking is more intense. When someone is in crisis, it's difficult for them to see alternatives to suicide because their mindset is overly pessimistic. Having a plan can help identify multiple options your partner can use to reduce their distress and minimize the likelihood of a suicide attempt. Safety planning doesn't close the door to suicide entirely but diverts your partner from these thoughts, allowing them to consider other options. It helps you buy time and keeps your partner safe until the suicidal thoughts diminish and the door closes.

TRY THIS: CREATING A SAFETY PLAN

Collaborate with your partner to make a safety plan. Do this when things are relatively calm and your partner's suicidal thinking isn't too intense. Here are the steps to consider and write down:

1. ***Warning signs.*** This is the alert system, much like the extreme weather alerts described earlier. Work with your partner to outline signs that indicate they are really stressed out or in a state of crisis. What thoughts do they have when this occurs? What situations tend to trigger a crisis? What behaviors do they exhibit? Are there physical sensations or

emotions that precede suicidal thinking that they should be aware of? For example, is your partner thinking of harming themself? Do they indicate that they wish they were dead or that you would be better off without them? Do they feel like a burden? Do they feel that their distress and pain are unbearable and will never go away?

2. ***Reasons for living.*** Are there things your partner looks forward to or that give them meaning or pleasure? Ask your partner what they think is worth living for. It might be you, your kids, a pet, their family. It is possible that your partner is so depressed that they can't think of any reason to live. If that is the case, try to see what used to give your partner a reason to live. You could even ask what reasons a friend or someone they admire would give. Just because it is difficult for your partner to come up with reasons to live doesn't mean that those reasons are not there. Keep trying.

3. ***Distraction and coping strategies.*** List some activities that might help divert your partner from suicidal thoughts and on to something else. Try to come up with a list of five different activities your partner could do when feeling this way—things that would give them a sense of pleasure or mastery. It could involve drawing, listening to music, going for a walk, journaling, or breathing exercises. If their emotions are intense and they have a desire to harm themself, you could try having your partner hold a piece of ice in their hand. Although this can be painful after a while, it is one way they might be able to distract themself without causing physical harm.

Ideally, you would want to list things that are active and engage your partner rather than passive things like watching television. But if watching a show does the trick, add it to the list. Even better, your partner might consider doing things that are distracting but also involve some form of social connection, like going out for coffee, going to the gym, or meeting someone for a stroll.

You could also list things that your partner has tried and found helpful in the past or strategies they think might work in the future.

4. ***Contacts.*** Come up with a list of people your partner can speak with in a crisis. It is often helpful if these contacts also know about the safety plan and how they can best help. If no one comes to mind, which is sometimes the case, you can skip this step.

5. ***Professionals.*** Include a list of professionals that your partner could contact if these steps have not minimized their risk and your partner is still in crisis. This could include their psychologist or other licensed

mental health professional, their family doctor, or a local crisis helpline. In the United States and Canada, you could also list 988 (the national Suicide and Crisis Lifeline), a free and confidential service that is available 24/7. They could also text HOME to 741741, which connects them at any hour to a free crisis counselor through the Crisis Text Line.

This plan can be written on a 3" × 5" index card or typed into your partner's notes app on their phone. By addressing each of these steps thoughtfully and with compassion, you can play a crucial role in reducing the risk of suicide and supporting your loved one during this difficult time.

If you suspect that your partner is in danger of acting on their thoughts, the best thing you can do is take them to a hospital or mental health facility or call 911. In some cities, there are mobile crisis units that will come to your home to assess the risk of danger and make recommendations for next steps, including going to the emergency room. This can be hard, and they may be angry at you for pushing this, but it's a way to keep them safe when things get really bad.

Involuntary Admission

If your partner shows signs that they are likely to harm themself, it is incredibly important to take this seriously. The first thing you should do is make sure they are safe. If your partner has talked about suicide or shown drastic changes in behavior—like giving away belongings, suddenly withdrawing from loved ones, making a plan, acquiring harmful items, or expressing severe feelings of hopelessness—it's critical to intervene. Stay with them if possible; do not leave them alone.

There may be times when your partner is at risk of harming themself or others and you need to make the difficult decision to have them hospitalized against their will. This can be excruciating and might temporarily damage the trust your partner has in you.

Tricia regularly encouraged her partner, Justin, to seek professional help, but he adamantly refused, insisting that he could handle it on his own. Over the previous couple of days, she noticed that Justin's behavior had changed dramatically. One evening, things quickly took a dark turn. "I can't handle this anymore. I'm done," Justin admitted. Tricia was shocked by the gravity of Justin's comment and started to tremble. In addition to feeling frightened, she was deeply hurt and disappointed. Tricia had worked so hard to support Justin and hoped he would soon turn a corner. She worried he was now in danger of harming himself.

After some heated discussion, Justin finally agreed to let Tricia drive him to the hospital. When they arrived, the psychiatric team evaluated Justin and concluded that he needed inpatient care. Justin was confused and angry with Tricia and the hospital staff. He refused to understand why he couldn't just get an adjustment to his medication and go home.

The days following Justin's admission were long and incredibly difficult for Tricia. She missed Justin but, more than that, she felt like a traitor and was overwhelmed with guilt. Tricia replayed scenarios in her mind, repeatedly questioning how things could have reached this point and whether her support had been sufficient. Deep down, Tricia knew this was the right decision, but there would be a lot of work ahead helping Justin improve and processing the complex aftermath of emotions they both experienced.

Obviously, it would be best (and easier for everyone involved) if your partner were willing to come to this decision on their own. Try to approach them with compassion and understanding. If you feel that they are in danger, try to talk to your partner about why you believe they need professional care, including hospitalization. It is important to be nonjudgmental and avoid making them feel as though they're being punished or have failed. Let them know you care and want to help them through the process. If they are still resistant, explain that you are worried about their well-being and need to call for help. They may be very distressed and angry at you for coming to this conclusion. They may feel misunderstood, stigmatized, or even betrayed. You can't control their feelings, but you can validate them and continue to express that you're acting out of care for their safety. It's important to remain calm and empathic, while staying firm in your resolve to keep them safe. Stay strong. Remind yourself that you are doing what is in their best interest even if they don't see it at the time.

Although the laws differ from country to country (and from state to state, or province to province), they generally converge on the criteria that the person may be involuntarily admitted to a hospital if they are a danger to themself or others due to a mental disorder. This can be initiated by a police officer, a physician, a psychologist, or a family member. If this process is initiated, your partner would typically be assessed in an emergency department or psychiatric facility. There is a period (usually 72 hours) to determine whether your partner should be admitted to the hospital against their will. Usually there is a requirement that the individual subject to involuntary admission be informed of their rights, have access to legal counsel, and may challenge the decision through an independent review process.

Dealing with involuntary admission can be incredibly difficult. It involves a delicate balance between protecting your partner's well-being and respecting their autonomy. If your partner is admitted involuntarily, continue to be there for them throughout the process. They may have feelings of shame, fear, or anger after being hospitalized. Although you may have to wait until the dust settles, try to help them work through these emotions and let them know that you are there for them. You may also experience feelings of guilt, sadness, or frustration. Make sure you prioritize your own mental and emotional well-being as well during this time. You may want to reach out friends, a mental health professional, or a support group to help you through this challenging time.

Managing Expectations

Recovery from depression is often not a simple, linear process. Your partner will experience good days and bad days. There will be successes and setbacks. It's important to manage your expectations and come to grips with the fact that there is no quick fix for depression. In most cases depression will improve within a year and sometimes as quickly as a few months. The more your partner is willing to engage in behavioral activation and changing thinking, the quicker they will respond. However, for others, the process may take longer. It might require ongoing treatment, modifications in approaches, and new strategies over time.

Acknowledging that your partner's symptoms may not improve quickly, even with considerable effort on their part, might help you offer continued compassion and support. Learning to accept that this may be a long journey with periods of both progress and frustration will help you stay the course. Be patient with your partner and with yourself and try to find hope and optimism.

One way to stay optimistic and hopeful is to focus on the small victories. When your partner is in the depths of depression, it can be hard for them to see even the smallest improvements. Depression imposes a dark cloud over everything. However, you may also miss seeing change because you are exhausted, frustrated, and distressed yourself. Making an effort to focus on the small things that are signs of improvement, like consistently getting out of bed or being able to engage in a conversation, can help you both shift the focus away from what *isn't* working to what is.

Another way to keep hope alive is to rely on your social support networks. As a partner, it can be helpful to know that you are not alone in your struggles. Reaching out to family and friends can provide a sense of support and might help you see things from a different angle. Support groups for loved ones of individuals with depression or even online communities can also be helpful. They provide an opportunity to connect with individuals who are wrestling with some of the same things you are, understand the journey, and provide both emotional support and practical advice. You may also consider seeing a psychologist or other mental health provider yourself. Bouncing ideas off an expert and learning strategies for maintaining your own well-being can be beneficial. Although there is no magic bullet for depression, that doesn't mean progress is impossible. There is hope for change, even in the toughest circumstances. Stay strong.

When the bulk of your energy and focus is on your partner's well-being, it's easy to forget about yourself. Ensuring that your needs are being met and engaging in routines that promote self-care and help you recharge are also important. The next section of the book focuses on just that.

PART TWO

Supporting Yourself

8

Making Sense of Your Feelings and Tending to Your Needs

Kristen loved Mark, but every day she felt more resentment. Mark responded to his depression by isolating himself and retreating from everyone and everything. Even the kids started to ask about their dad, wondering why he never wanted to play or what made him so serious all the time. Kristen worried about how the kids were coping with all of this and that it would impact them negatively.

After 12 years of marriage, Kristen felt like a single mom. The responsibilities she and Mark once shared now fell squarely on her shoulders. She wanted to support Mark and tried to buffer the children from the fallout, so she kept pushing herself. Kristen assumed responsibility for everything—getting the kids ready for school, dropping them off, picking them up, taking them to and from soccer practices and dance rehearsals, preparing meals, cleaning the house, and doing the laundry. She had no downtime. No time for herself. She was exhausted.

What made it especially difficult was that Kristen felt completely alone. Her social life had all but vanished. Kristen knew that getting out with friends would be good for her, but she kept declining invitations. She needed to be home for Mark and the kids. In a sense, she was also protecting Mark. Kristen knew that she would be tempted to vent about Mark and thought it wouldn't be fair to him. Her friends eventually stopped reaching out because Kristen always had some excuse. She was either too busy or too tired.

She tried to be patient and to understand that the depression was not Mark's fault, but she was angry. It all seemed so unjust. Everything had become her responsibility whereas Mark barely got out of bed each day.

Although each person's story is unique, most struggle personally when their partner is depressed. As the depression lingers or worsens, you may experience a mix of wildly different and seemingly contradictory emotions, feelings that may be hard to understand, process, or deal with. Or, like Kristen, you might have gotten to the point where your feelings are no longer conflicted—there's just anger, resentment, and bitterness. Perhaps you're grieving the loss of companionship with your partner or having difficulties communicating honestly with them. Wanting to share your true feelings without hurting your partner may leave you feeling like you're always walking on eggshells. The energy spent caring for your partner and managing the added responsibilities may have left you depleted, starting to consider whether your relationship is still worth fighting for.

This chapter will help you work through some of these complex issues. To be sure, there are no easy answers. However, by recognizing that it's okay to feel conflicted, learning to manage these emotions, and taking steps to care for your own well-being, you will be in a better place to help yourself (and your partner) along the way.

Dealing with Conflicting Emotions

Living with someone who is depressed can take an emotional and physical toll on you and begin to color your perception of your partner. Some of the emotions you're wrestling with might be difficult to reconcile in your mind. For example, you might feel love and compassion for your partner but, at the same time, feel frustration and resentment toward them. These feelings might bubble up over time because you feel as though the relationship has become one-sided or your partner is emotionally distant or irritable. Although pulling far more of the weight in the relationship and day-to-day responsibilities may have felt acceptable when your partner first experienced depression, it can start to eat at you over time.

Another tension might be the desire to help versus feeling unappreciated. You may be working hard to support your partner with patience, kindness, and gentleness, and yet these efforts seem futile or ignored. Your partner may be irritable and lash out or withdraw from you. You may be left wondering why you're dedicating yourself to helping them. You also may struggle with the fact that you understand that depression isn't your partner's fault and experience empathy for them while also feeling surges of anger at being unappreciated.

Feeling exhausted and having trouble seeing the light at the end of the tunnel only serves to exacerbate this turmoil.

This is a complex emotional landscape where feelings of love, empathy, and care often coexist with frustration, anger, and resentment. Sometimes one side wins out more than the other. When thinking begins to shift toward more negative feelings about your partner, guilt and despair often result. You may scold yourself that you *should* be exclusively loving and supporting them. This is an example of the "should" statements mentioned in Chapter 6, and they don't make you a bad partner. In fact, considerable research has demonstrated that these responses are fairly typical.

TRY THIS: REFLECTING ON YOUR EMOTIONS

Take some time to reflect on your emotions. Do some of the conflicting emotions resonate with you? Are you also experiencing some of these seemingly contradictory emotions? What other emotions do you feel?

Try to recognize your feelings and validate them. They don't make you a bad partner. They also don't necessarily mean that you're giving up hope entirely. You aren't alone. Having conflicting emotions is quite common among people who are partnered with someone who is experiencing depression. As strange as it might seem, your feelings toward your partner don't have to be good *or* bad; they can be both good *and* bad or neutral.

What you want to do, however, is understand your emotions and try to manage them so that you feel better about your role as a caregiver and can maintain your sanity. It's a frustrating and exhausting roller coaster, and you may need to grieve what you've lost (temporarily) in your relationship. You may need to vent your emotions with a friend. You may need to take a break to meet your own needs.

Will My Real Partner Please Stand Up?

Another feeling you might be experiencing is a loss of companionship. At one time your partner was the first person you turned to to share positive news or when you needed support over bad news. Now, instead of getting a sense of vibrancy and passion with your partner, there is distance. It's so painful to sit right next to the person you had every intention of sharing your life with only to feel alone in your relationship. You want your partner back!

Depression often leads to emotional withdrawal, making it difficult to maintain the connection and companionship you once had. Many people who have partners with depression report a loss of the partnership, where emotional and physical intimacy become a distant memory. This often leads to feelings of loneliness and despair. You might also be feeling as though you can't get close to your partner. You tell your partner that you love them, and they may be unresponsive, unable to reciprocate. It guts you. Communication, which used to be so easy, is now negative or nonexistent.

Although it's easier said than done, try to recognize that your partner isn't trying to be distant or withdrawn. The behavior is more a reflection of the weight and magnitude of what they are going through than how they feel about you. Viewing it as unintentional might not ease your pain but may at least make you feel less lost.

When you're feeling lonely and sad, try to push against the urge to shut down. Maintaining an open line of communication may never be more important than it is right now. Without blaming, talk to your partner about what's going on for you and how the emotional distance is impacting you. You might say something like "I miss connecting with you. I feel as though we've become more distant with each other lately, and I want to work on that. Would you be open to that?" Then come up with a plan for how the two of you might reconnect. Start small and try to have realistic expectations. Rather than expecting your partner to immediately return to the way they were before depression, acknowledge that the closeness you desire may take time to rebuild. You don't want to set yourself up for further disappointment.

Then try to foster a sense of connection through baby steps. Even small gestures can go a long way, and your partner will be more likely to come around and eventually reciprocate if you are consistent with your attempts at connection. A gentle touch, a cup of tea, a back rub. Spend quality time together even if it's difficult and unrewarding.

My Social Life Is on Hold!

Many people feel as though their social lives are put on hold when their partner has depression. There may be several contributing factors, but you might be experiencing one or more of the following common responses.

Your Partner Doesn't Have the Desire or Energy to Socialize

People with depression often find social interaction draining and burdensome. If you were used to getting out together with others, this may come as a real shock to you. You may feel increasingly restricted and isolated. If so, consider revisiting Chapter 5 and seeing if you can slowly start to help your partner reengage bit by bit with behavioral activation. Having an honest, but gentle, conversation with your partner about how this is important to you, good for their mental health, and beneficial to your relationship might also help. If your partner is up for it, you could try to introduce some low-pressure get-together or invite a friend over to your place to keep the social interaction minimal but still fulfilling.

Sheila felt resistance from Greg every time she suggested doing something social. Their plans always had to be on Greg's terms. If he suggested something, he was likely to proceed, but if she recommended the same thing, he'd resist. Even when Sheila suggested they get together with old friends whose kids were the same age as theirs, or just for a quick drink out, Greg would invariably decline, stating, "I don't know. I'm such a loser. I won't have anything to say."

For his 50th birthday, Greg didn't want to have a party, but Sheila decided to tell a few friends, "If you just happened to show up on the doorstep and knock, we'll invite you in and say a quick hello," as a surprise for her husband. She knew if someone came to the door, Greg wouldn't turn them away. And it turned out that Greg liked it. It lifted his mood, and he appreciated that these people came over and hung out for a bit.

It's also important not to neglect your own relationships. Having a social life isn't entirely dependent on your partner joining you. It may require having to suddenly learn to interact with other friends and couples on your own, but it's important to ensure that you maintain social connections.

You're Too Exhausted Yourself

Do you find yourself avoiding seeing friends and family because you're exhausted from taking on all the responsibilities involved in supporting your partner? After working all day, making dinner, doing the dishes, and helping your kids with their homework and bedtime routine, you may have no more gas in the tank (or to be more environmentally friendly, juice in the battery).

This loss of a social life can be problematic. Now, more than ever, you need support.

As difficult as it might seem to muster the drive, it's important to continue to get together with others and ensure you have a social life. This is critical not only to give yourself a break and replenish your resources, but also because it can be fun. Getting together with others might also allow you to share your problems and get support yourself. Research consistently demonstrates that social connection is critical for our mental and physical health.

You Feel Guilty Leaving Your Partner Home Alone

This is a tough dilemma. It's natural to feel torn between wanting to support your partner and the need to maintain your own well-being. However, your needs matter too! Taking care of yourself is not selfish. You can't be on call 24/7 when your partner is struggling. Not only will having a social life help you feel better, but it will also refill your tank so that you can continue the hard work of supporting your partner. Your social life is part of maintaining your well-being, and this balance can help you be there for your partner in a more sustainable way. Acknowledge your guilt, but don't let it control your decisions. Guilt is an emotion that says, "I've done something wrong." You haven't. You aren't abandoning your partner.

In some instances, your partner may lay a guilt trip on you. Don't let that dictate what you do. Have an open conversation with your partner and express that you want to be there for them but also need some time to recharge.

You're Embarrassed about Your Partner's Depression

You may avoid friends because you don't know what to say when others ask about your partner. Perhaps you are tired of making up excuses for why your partner hasn't shown up to social events. It may be too difficult to admit that your partner is struggling with depression, or you want to respect your partner's privacy. You might fear that people won't understand what you're going through, know what to say or, worse, will make disparaging or unhelpful comments. This, in turn, might lead you to withdraw from social support.

In this case you might want to remind yourself that depression is more common than you think. When someone asks me what I do for work, invariably they tell me stories about their own, their partner's, or some family member or friend who suffers from depression. Depression affects all of us! Most people can relate to struggles with mental health in some form.

Fortunately, the stigma associated with mental health is decreasing and many people are open to talking about their experiences. You may feel as though you're alone, but you're not. Obviously, you'll want to be selective, sharing your experiences with people you trust and have a good relationship with. They are more likely to listen and be supportive. If you aren't sure it's a good idea to bring it up, start with small disclosures and gauge how others respond. Instead of making the focus on your partner's depression, think about sharing your own challenges: "It's been difficult to know how best to support my partner through their depression. I've been feeling quite isolated and overwhelmed by it all." Although you want to be mindful of protecting your partner's privacy, sharing some of your experiences with close friends or family can allow you to get the support you need. So take a risk—you might be surprised. There is no shame in what you or your partner are going through.

You might also consider joining a self-help group that can provide support and helpful feedback from others who are going through similar struggles. This will also help you realize that you're not alone and provide you with a new social network. If you're not able to access social support in person, online forums and communities (like Reddit or HealthUnlocked) can be another way to connect with people who understand what you're going through. Be careful, however, not to buy into everything you read. Sometimes these forums can spread misinformation as well.

I'm Walking on Eggshells

Another common feeling is the need to mask your feelings or guard your tongue when your partner is depressed. Sometimes it feels as though you're "walking on eggshells," worried that you might say something that will trigger them, instigate an argument, set them off, or be hurtful. So you resort to hiding your feelings, tiptoeing around.

This was Stephon's strategy. Irene had been struggling with depression for months, and although he loved Irene and was genuinely concerned for her, Stephon felt more and more resentful that his own needs weren't being met. Instead of expressing them openly, Stephon learned to hide his true feelings, pretending that everything was okay and choosing silence over conflict. His relationship felt fake. Whenever they interacted, Stephon would just smile at Irene and be supportive, pretending everything was okay. This left him feeling empty and alone. Meanwhile, Irene had no clue this was Stephon's experience. Over time, his unspoken thoughts became more difficult to suppress.

The concern about triggering or upsetting your partner by sharing your feelings is palpable, especially when they are emotionally fragile. Yet not sharing your feelings can be more destructive in the long run. It's not fair to you, and it's not fair to your partner. Trying to maintain an open line of communication, although difficult, is important. Both of you need to feel safe to share what you're going through.

The first thing you can do is recognize that depression impacts the way people react emotionally. Your partner doesn't have their normal emotion regulation skills, leaving them vulnerable to perceiving comments as critical or hurtful even when they weren't meant that way. Thinking is skewed negatively when someone is depressed. As a result, your partner's reaction may be out of proportion because of their thinking traps (see Chapter 6). They may personalize, catastrophize, mind-read, or view your comments through a lens of all-or-nothing thinking. This doesn't mean you should bury your feelings. It just means that how and when you approach what's on your mind may make a difference. Think about the timing. Your message is more likely to be received in the way you intend it at a time when things aren't already heated. Also, try to recognize that your partner's reactions may speak more about the depression than about you. This might help you bring things up with a dose of empathy rather than avoiding them out of fear.

Do your best to ensure that your comments aren't coming across as judgmental or critical, but be prepared for the fallout—regardless of what you say, or how kind and gentle you are, your partner might interpret your message through a negative filter. Your partner is vulnerable and likely afraid of being judged or criticized or rejected. Acknowledge your feelings and express them while being mindful that depression will impact how the message is received.

Try to validate what your partner is going through, but be honest about what you're experiencing. Your partner's depression may cause them to react strongly, but remind yourself it's not your fault. You aren't responsible for controlling or managing your partner's emotions. There is no perfect way to do this and there may be some backlash or hurt feelings, but try to recognize that you can work through this and that avoiding will only make things worse.

I Didn't Sign Up for This!

Especially if your partner is severely depressed, you may find yourself overwhelmed by the new role you're playing, the new responsibilities that you're taking on alone. In addition to providing emotional support and taking care of the household and family, there may be added financial pressures, especially if your partner can no longer work, is on short- or long-term disability, or needs to cut back on work hours. The pressure can be intense, and you might be thinking "I didn't sign up for this! I feel as though I'm never off duty. This isn't fair."

You're right; you didn't sign up for this. And you have a right to feel frustrated, tired, or even resentful. But try not to get stuck in thinking that you've been forced into this, you have no control, or this will never end. You'll only end up feeling more depleted and angrier. Take time to acknowledge and validate your feelings, reach out to people you trust for help and support, and try to view this predicament as temporary. Remind yourself that this is brutal, but you're doing the best you can. Focus on what you can control—how you respond to this difficult situation and what you can do to keep your own sanity. Your partner's depression won't last forever. Although it is super difficult to see when you are in the thick of it all, try to remind yourself why you got in this relationship in the first place. Depression has changed your relationship dynamics and turned your world upside down, but the person you fell in love with is still there and they can improve. With your help and support, and the assistance of professionals, they will be more likely to climb out of this hole and you will get your life and your relationship back.

What about My Own Mental Health?

Let's face it. What you're dealing with is incredibly difficult and likely triggers numerous emotions for you. You may experience any combination of being overwhelmed, sad, anxious, worried, angry, frustrated, resentful, or bitter. Supporting a partner with depression can take a toll on you too. More than 40% of partners of individuals with depression end up feeling so devastated and distressed that they need professional help themselves. More than one-third of caregivers of individuals with bipolar disorder report high levels of depressive symptoms. Living with someone who struggles with depression can significantly impact your own mood.

So much of your time and emotional energy has been devoted to your partner that you may not have given much thought to your own mental health and well-being. Many people who support partners with depression experience caregiver burnout, a period of physical, emotional, and mental exhaustion that can occur when you're supporting someone. It's so easy to forget or neglect to take care of yourself while you're taking care of everything else.

Caregivers who experience burnout may feel tired, stressed, withdrawn, anxious, and depressed. And neglecting your own well-being can increase bitterness toward your partner, put a strain on your relationship, and also negatively impact your partner's depression.

If you find that your stress levels have hit an all-time high, you may want to reach out to a mental health care provider, such as a psychologist, for individual therapy. They will be able to help you work through your feelings and generate ways to better handle your stress. A therapist can also help you figure out some logistics, like managing your role as caregiver, navigating concerns with your children, or working through financial issues. Seeing a therapist might also be beneficial for understanding and improving the interactions you have with your partner. They can also help you gain some control over what often seems like an uncontrollable situation.

Couple therapy is another option to consider. Couple therapy can help improve your relationship satisfaction, reduce the emotional burden you may be experiencing, understand the impact that your partner's depression is having on your relationship, improve communication, and develop strategies for managing emotional distress. More information about couple therapy is provided in Chapter 15.

Should I Stay or Go?

Another internal conflict you may experience is the desire to support your partner on one hand and to escape on the other. Fantasies like going on a vacation getaway by yourself, taking an emotional leave of absence, or leaving the relationship entirely are not uncommon. Having such thoughts doesn't mean you aren't committed to your partner. It may be a signal that you're feeling trapped by the endless demands on you and need to protect your own mental health.

Take some time to think about your relationship and your motivations. If you had a good relationship before your partner experienced depression—one characterized by mutual love and respect—your relationship may be worth fighting for. If significant relationship problems existed before your partner's depression, it may be even more difficult to bounce back from this and leaving may be the best option. What drew you to your partner initially? Are there qualities you still see in your partner that you know are there but perhaps colored or numbed by depression? If so, you may want to fight for getting them back. If you can't remember what attracted you to your partner or if your partner's depression has become the sole focus of the relationship and no emotional connection exists, you may consider leaving. There's no easy answer here.

Sometimes, for the sake of your own mental health and well-being, leaving the relationship is the best option. Before you go too far down that path, however, you will want to be confident that you have done everything you could to save the relationship. You don't want to make a hasty decision now only to live with guilt or regret later because you've second-guessed whether you could have done more or things could have improved. Have you consulted with friends? Have you spoken openly with your partner about your needs? Have you worked through some of these issues with a mental health professional? Have you tried couple therapy? If all these options have been tried and you are still stuck, it may be time to reevaluate whether you would be better off going. This decision will, of course, need to align with your own personal or religious convictions. Some of you may have taken seriously the vow of "in sickness and in health, till death do us part."

Is your partner working on their depression either through therapy, with medication, or via self-help resources? Are there any signs of improvement? If they are committed to actively working to get better and you are both able to communicate and work together, it may be worth giving it more time to see how things unfold. On the other hand, if your partner is unwilling to seek treatment or there is a long period of time when they have not tried to work with you to improve the relationship, you might need to consider leaving for your own sake.

Another consideration is whether staying in the relationship is severely impacting your own mental or physical health. If you are constantly drained and unable to support your partner *and* take care of your own emotional needs, it may be time to consider leaving. As well, if your partner's depression is leading to an unhealthy relationship where you're both suffering, your relationship is probably unsustainable. If there is emotional neglect or manipulation, or physical abuse in the relationship, seek professional support and consider leaving for your own safety and mental health. Your own safety and well-being must come first.

The severity of your partner's depression or threats (like revealing suicidal thoughts or intentions) should also not be the reason you stay. Suicidal threats need to be taken seriously, but sticking around because you are concerned for your partner's safety may only make you resent them or further worsen your relationship. Although you can help to ensure their safety, you are not responsible for your partner's well-being or their choices.

Of course, every relationship has rough and dry patches, and a partner's depression is not easy to manage. That doesn't necessarily mean that the relationship should be terminated. However, if you believe you've given it your best shot, and there is no glimmer of hope that these issues will improve, you might want to think about a trial or permanent separation. You deserve happiness and fulfillment too.

9

Understanding Your Responsibility

Many people question whether they played a role in causing their partner's depression, especially when the condition first appears. They may wonder later if how they're handling this new situation is making the depression worse. And, as discussed in the preceding chapter, the question of how much responsibility a nondepressed partner should take for all the needs of the person with depression, the family, and the household comes up regularly. It's important to know where your responsibility begins and ends so you don't get overwhelmed by guilt or resentment. Let's start with cause.

Is My Partner's Depression My Fault?

As discussed in Chapter 1, it's impossible to determine with any level of certainty what caused your partner's depression. There are numerous potential origins of depression that involve a complex combination of biological, psychological, and social factors. It's only natural, however, to wonder whether your relationship is the problem. Relationship distress may in fact be a factor, but which is the cause and which the effect? Depression can cause relationship distress just as much as relationship distress contributes to depression. It's also important to remember that it takes two to tango. Even if relationship distress was one of the contributors to your partner's depression, you weren't necessarily the sole cause of that distress.

The truth is that depression typically isn't anyone's fault—not yours to own and not your partner's. It's usually not about what you did or didn't do. The best thing you can do in this instance is accept that you won't ever know the cause(s) of your partner's depression and direct your attention, instead, to what you have control over now and what you can change going forward.

It's not that reflecting on the past isn't helpful. It can be. But you want to "visit the graveyard, not pitch a tent there." If you feel so inclined, go ahead and think about what you could have done differently, how you may not have been as present or kind or loving as you would have liked. Just as understanding history can help society address and sidestep future issues by not repeating mistakes, let this review inform what you can do now and in the future. Ruminating about what you could have changed and dwelling on the past, however, won't help you or your partner move forward.

TRY THIS: RESPONSIBILITY PIE

Take a moment or two to think about how much you believe you have contributed to your partner's depression. What percentage of responsibility do you think you own?

Let's work through this feeling by creating what's called a *responsibility pie*. If you're willing, grab a writing instrument and some paper and draw a big circle. Now fill in the portion of the pie you feel responsible for. How much do you believe you have contributed to your partner's depression? Is it 70%? 80%? More? Less? Fill in how much you think you are responsible.

Let's say you feel 80% responsible. If that's the case, your responsibility pie would look something like this:

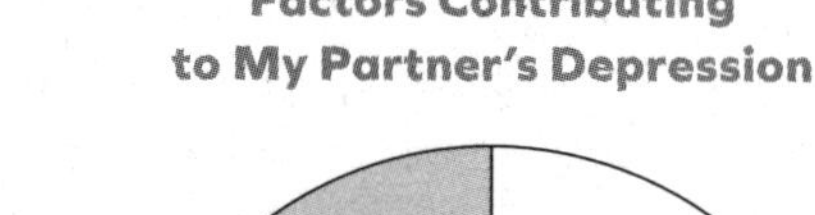

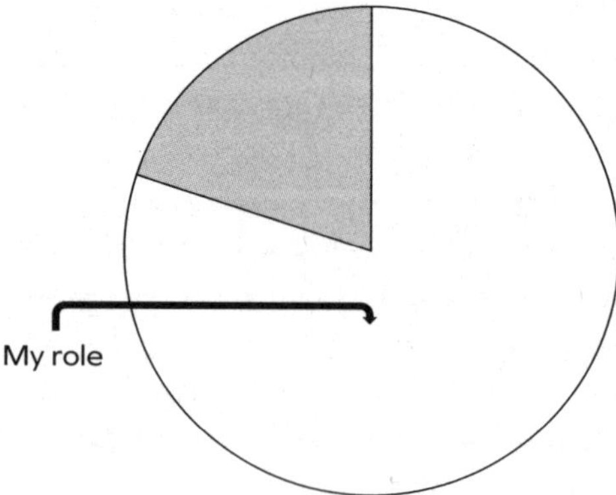

Now, on the same or a different page, draw another circle. This time, rather than considering your contribution, think first about all the different things that may have impacted your partner's depression. It could be stress at work, financial concerns, difficulties with other relationships, avoidance behavior, biological factors, family history of depression, social isolation, history of trauma, losing a friend or an important role—any number of things. Try to include as many factors as you think are reasonable and assign a percentage to each of them. For example, if you thought that negative thinking, chronic back pain, social isolation, work stress, and avoidance contributed 25%, 20%, 15%, 15%, and 15%, respectively, fill each of those in the circle. Don't worry about the exact percentages; just try to estimate. In this case the responsibility pie would look like this:

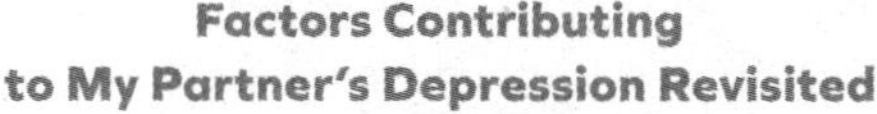

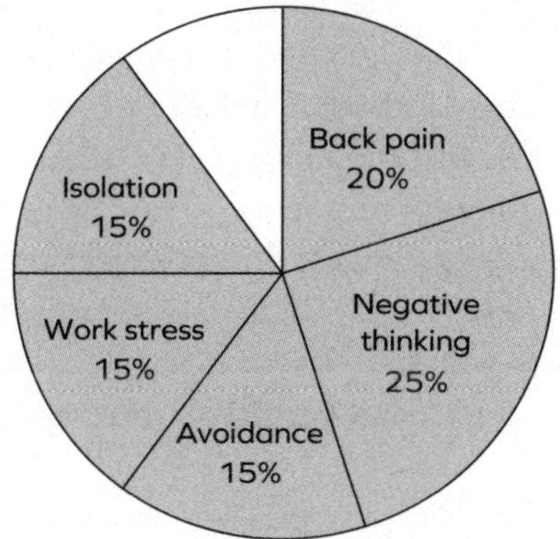

Once you do this exercise, you might come to realize that there are many variables that have influenced your partner's depression and that this isn't all your fault. In this example, your responsibility would be 10%, not 80% as you initially felt.

Rather than focusing on the cause of depression or who is to blame, having a discussion on what is happening now and what you can do to help improve things may be more beneficial. For instance, you could ask your partner if there is anything you are doing currently that may be affecting their stress or depression.

It's also possible that your partner doesn't realize their impact on you. This may be important to discuss at some point as well. For now, see what you can do but try not to internalize or personalize your partner's experience. Yes, depression and relationship stress do often go hand in hand, but this doesn't mean you're responsible for your partner's depression or their recovery. This is a journey that they must take—you can be there to support them along the way, but they need to take the necessary steps.

Hopefully the responsibility pie has helped you recognize that you are not at fault for your partner's depression. If you have found this exercise helpful, you might want to try it for other areas in your life where you feel too much responsibility. Although this exercise might best be completed on your own, you could also have a discussion with your partner about the responsibility pie, if you think that's warranted or would be helpful.

Emily had wrestled with Paul's depression for many months. Now she felt like she was losing him and somehow to blame for how Paul was feeling. "Maybe I'm the problem," she told herself. "Maybe my behavior has created negative ripples that have impacted Paul's depression. What if I'm not doing enough? I've been so focused on work that I might have neglected our relationship for a while. And also because of work, I've been kind of impatient with him lately."

At first Emily believed she was 75% responsible for Paul's depression, but that felt like an exaggeration, so she decided to consider her piece of the pie—the part she was responsible for—last and started to make a mental list of other possible contributions to her partner's depression:

- Paul had lost his job in the recent downsizing of his company. Even though the layoff wasn't his fault, it lowered his self-confidence and he had stopped submitting resumes after looking for work online for several weeks and getting no interview invitations.
- Paul had also started to avoid getting together with friends. He used to be so active after work and would regularly meet up with a group of guys for pickup basketball or just to hang out. All of this came to a grinding halt after being laid off, perhaps because Paul was ashamed or embarrassed about being out of work.

Emily used the responsibility pie technique to allocate responsibility for Paul's depression, as shown in the figure on page 127, and realized that she was not responsible for Paul's depression nor was the onus on her to "fix" him.

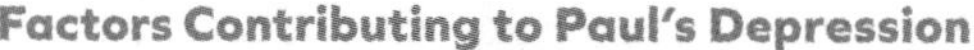

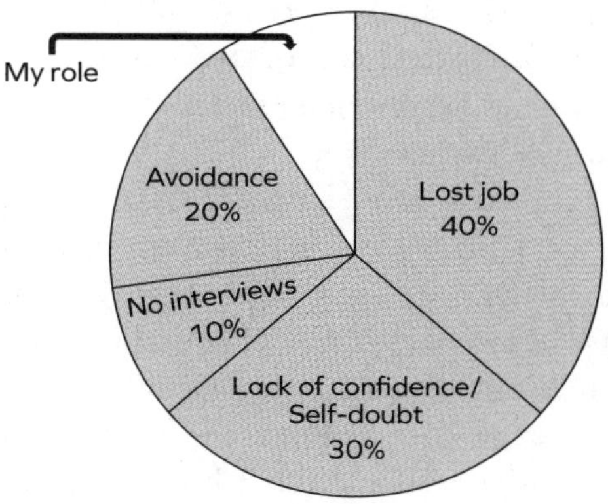

Challenging Self-Blame

Recognizing that you're not solely responsible for your partner's depression is not simple. This feeling may bubble up occasionally and sometimes percolate for too long. It's so easy to fall into the trap of questioning yourself. *If only I had seen the signs earlier. If only I had supported them more. I should have pushed them to get help. If only I hadn't gotten so frustrated and angry.* When you have these kinds of thoughts, it may be helpful to complete a responsibility pie. It can also be beneficial to pay attention to your thoughts and evaluate them with evidence (see Chapter 6). For example, asking yourself, "What would my friend say if they knew I had this thought?" or "What would I say to my friend if I knew they were thinking this?" can help you see things a little more objectively.

Responding When Your Partner Blames You

Sometimes blame comes not from you but directly from your partner. And it can sting. When people are depressed, they sometimes look outside of themselves to find the source of their unhappiness. They desperately want to change how they are feeling but don't know how and end up blaming the person closest to them. They may say things that they normally wouldn't, lash out at you, or push you away. There may be days when you can't seem to say or do anything right and feel like you're just a dumping ground for all their negativity. You might not even be sure who you are dealing with on a given day.

Sara had been with Cheryl for six years. Cheryl had experienced recurrent depression off and on since her early teens, and her most recent episode, two years into the relationship, seemed to last the longest and was punctuated with anxiety and agitation. Cheryl would periodically lash out at Sara for no apparent reason. And Sara was hurt by it.

One afternoon, Sara met a friend for coffee and described the situation: "I'm not sure who I'm dealing with," she exclaimed. "Is it Dr. Jekyll or Ms. Hyde? If I'm dealing with Dr. Jekyll, our days are pretty good and there is no turmoil or blame. But I brace myself when I'm dealing with Ms. Hyde and watch everything I say and do to avoid setting her off."

Sara's friend encouraged her to think about what was coming from Cheryl's depression and what was related to Cheryl as a person (her character, her personality) or the relationship itself: "Is that depression talking or is Cheryl just mean?" When depression or anxiety was driving Cheryl's behavior, Sara learned to take her comments with a grain of salt and not personalize them. For example, Sara would sometimes say to herself, *Cheryl doesn't mean what she's saying. She's just worked up right now. Her thinking is so negative she can't even see straight. I know that, deep down inside, she loves me. It's the depression talking. Cheryl will act differently when she starts to feel better.* Although Cheryl's comments were sometimes spiteful and insensitive, this self-talk helped Sara shake them off and attribute her remarks to the depression. This didn't mean that Sara was passive or simply put up with Cheryl's behavior. In fact, there were times when Sara would feel the need to defend herself and draw the line. However, framing it as part of the depression helped deescalate the situation and allowed Sara to not internalize Cheryl's statements or take them too personally.

Another helpful strategy is to remove yourself from the situation for a period to regroup and calm down. It can also be useful to recognize when your partner is just venting. Rather than taking it personally, distancing yourself mentally from the comments and chalking them up to the need to vent can help.

Yvonne had been married to George for over 30 years. Before the couple met, George had gone through a bad breakup and experienced his first episode of depression. However, things were good when he met Yvonne, and it wasn't until five years into their marriage that George experienced additional episodes. Yvonne got to the point where she was constantly feeling miserable. George would get into his "funks" and complain about everyone and everything. Sometimes he would blurt out, "You guys don't love me" or "Everybody hates me." Yvonne felt like she was doing everything wrong, and her own mood got worse each time George hurled these biting daggers. George would occasionally threaten suicide, which left Yvonne feeling even more helpless.

Yvonne eventually met up with a psychologist to figure out how best to work with George. When she described the situation, the psychologist asked, "Do you know when he's severely depressed versus when he just needs to vent? Because maybe in those moments, your job is to just listen. Let him vent and try not to take it personally." Yvonne was a little resistant and thought, "No. He shouldn't be saying those things!" But, after considering this suggestion more, Yvonne decided to try it out.

The first time Yvonne implemented this strategy, George was venting and saying all sorts of horrible things. Instead of absorbing these comments, Yvonne tried to be present and listen. Although the words that came out of George's mouth were like poison, Yvonne said to herself, "He's just venting." With this new perspective, Yvonne ended up reacting very differently to George's tirade. Almost mid-sentence, George noticed that Yvonne wasn't getting caught up in his rant. He stumbled on his words, paused, and looked perplexed. Yvonne said, "Sometimes you need to vent, and I just need to listen and let you vent." George could only respond with a "Huh."

Yvonne learned an important lesson. Previously, she would get pulled into a pattern of reacting to George's negativity and get worked up herself. This only made their interaction worse. By reappraising it as "venting," Yvonne was able to respond more calmly to George's behavior which, in turn, lessened the intensity of his outbursts.

Yvonne also learned another important lesson. George felt more validated when she explained to him what she was doing. She reported, "If I just didn't react, and the situation was sincerely bad for George, he would accuse me of not listening or think I don't care. But I explained to him that I was truly listening but letting him vent." This allowed George to be heard, and, at the same time, Yvonne didn't have to buy into it. She didn't have to try to fix it. She didn't overreact to it. "It wasn't me saying, 'No, I don't care about what you're saying, or I don't believe anything you say. You're full of shit.' It was me saying, 'Okay, I'm just going to sit here and listen.'" This helped turn things around, and George spiraled less than he would have had Yvonne gotten caught up in the turmoil.

There are also times when you need to be firm and stand up for yourself. For instance, Yvonne wouldn't allow George to walk all over her. There were times when Yvonne reached her limit and would say, "George, I know that you are depressed and really frustrated right now. But I am not the enemy here. You're moody and freaking out on me, and that's not cool. I need to be treated with respect."

Your needs are important too, and sometimes you need to call your partner out on inappropriate behavior. In a matter-of-fact tone, let them know that what they are saying (or how they're saying it) isn't right. Your partner is experiencing depression; they aren't clueless. Underneath the confusion and illogical mood shifts, they know when they're being hurtful. It's okay to let your partner know that they're out of line and need to stop treating you with malice and disrespect (see Chapter 13 for more tips on communication).

Sorting Out Blame

The only person in your relationship you have any control over is you. However, the way you respond can also impact your partner's responses positively or negatively. If blame is being dished out:

- Take a moment to evaluate whether you own any of the responsibility.
- Try to separate what might be due to your partner's depression versus their character or the relationship.
- See if you can temporarily remove yourself from the situation so that cooler heads can prevail.
- Allow your partner to vent without getting caught up in the whirlwind.
- Try not to personalize the insults, jabs, or negative comments.
- Stand up for yourself—your needs matter too.

How Do I Know If I'm Doing Too Much?

In Chapter 8 we discussed how much work can land in your lap when your partner is depressed. Responsibilities that used to be shared either become yours or don't get done. Partners (especially women of male partners with depression) tend to take on an exorbitant amount of the household responsibilities, including cooking, cleaning, childcare, and finances—all while working, being there for their loved one, supporting them in a caring way, and trying to show no signs of frustration or resentment.

Dealing with all these responsibilities can be overwhelming, especially when you're balancing your own emotions with the needs of your partner. It's tricky to know if you're doing too much. You want to be supportive, but you also need to take care of yourself.

Jadwiga wasn't sure how to balance meeting her own needs with supporting her husband, Antoni. Although they had been together for several years, Jadwiga was just beginning to make sense of the patterns the couple had fallen into and hadn't yet figured out what worked best. She did, however, finally realize that Antoni's recovery wasn't her responsibility: "I can't take care of his depression. That's up to him," she said. "It's in his camp. I will do what I can to support him, but, no matter how much I love him and want to help, I cannot take responsibility for his life." Yet Jadwiga was taking on more of the household responsibilities than she could handle and was exhausted. She decided to speak with Antoni about this issue and how to balance supporting him, managing day-to-day duties, and having at least some time to rest and recharge. At first Antoni wasn't open to having this conversation, but Jadwiga persisted. She mentioned that "changing the way things operate around here is important to me and will ultimately be helpful for you. We will confront your depression together, but we can't let it dictate our lives."

How much responsibility to take on is difficult to determine. Essentially, it boils down to what you are willing to do and how willing you are to do it. No one—not friends, family, or even professionals—can give you the "correct" answer. It depends on your own individual values and goals (see Chapter 14). How important is it for you to have your partner in your life? If it is fundamental, you might go to great lengths to help them. Someone who is committed to their partner and willing to stick it out, for example, might be willing to sacrifice quite a bit to help them overcome their depression and fight for the relationship. To them, the cost is steep, but it's worth the investment to help their partner and save the relationship. Another person may already be mentally checked out and on the cusp of calling it quits. This individual may be willing to support their partner, but to a lesser extent, and decide to put a time limit on how long they can sustain it. Others may be committed to their partner but nonetheless need to limit how much they do for their own sanity and mental health. Some individuals may be confused about where they land on this decision. They want to support their partner as much as they can but have doubts and may be teetering on the verge of giving up.

Think about where you fall on this continuum from being "all in" to being "almost out." Also, recognize that where you are now may be different than when your partner's depression began and may still change down the road. By picking up this book, you have at least demonstrated that you are willing to give it a solid effort. You may not be all in, but you're willing to give it a go.

I can't tell you what is best for you. That's a decision you need to reach yourself. What I can do is provide some things to think about and help you understand what's reasonable, what you are capable of, and where you might want to draw the line.

Your Partner's Recovery Is Ultimately Their Responsibility, Not Yours

Linda and Geoff were high school sweethearts. The couple dated for about a decade. When the relationship began, it was Linda who was having difficulties. She was in foster care and struggling in school. Here was this "normal" guy who seemed stable and came from a great family. But the trajectory changed over the years. Linda went from failing in school to excelling. Geoff, on the other hand, seemed to deteriorate, and by the end of high school, things started to fall apart for him. He began to experience all sorts of existential thoughts, like "What's the point? What am I going to do next?" Geoff felt as though everyone was moving forward and he was being left behind, stagnated. He continued to live with his mom. He smoked pot every day. And his mood got worse. He started waking up late, became withdrawn, and wouldn't answer Linda's calls. It got to the point where Geoff wasn't doing anything at all.

Linda encouraged Geoff to get help. And there were moments when Geoff would rally and seem to be motivated to change. But that would fade, and Linda ended up doing everything for Geoff. Meanwhile, her own needs were being neglected. This pattern went on for years—Linda would feel encouraged when Geoff expressed a desire to change. She would get incentivized to help. But it wouldn't be long before Geoff resorted to his old passive behavior. Linda assumed all responsibility. She would book appointments for Geoff. She'd write out a script of what to say to his doctor. She helped him with college applications and would give him recommendations about what he might want to do for a career. She would even assist Geoff with setting up a healthier daily schedule: "Right now, you're waking up at a different time every day. That must be really confusing for your body. What if you tried to wake up a little bit earlier at the same time every day and get out of the house for a bit?"

It was a long time before Linda realized that she was doing everything for Geoff. When he didn't follow through with the plans they made to help him feel better, Linda would feel resentful. "Why won't you just go to the doctor? Why won't you just take medication? Why don't you want to go to therapy? That's fine if you don't want to talk to somebody. Why won't you at least talk to your doctor about being put on some meds? Why am I the only one doing this?"

It got to the point where Linda had to do all the work to help Geoff or they were both going to end up at the bottom of an emotional pit. Linda eventually broke up with Geoff, but she continued to feel guilty for not being able to "fix" him. In retrospect, Linda understood that it wasn't her role to save Geoff. Geoff's decision to change (or not change) had to come from him.

It's common to feel distressed when the person you love has changed. Your interactions may have been stripped of their luster. Now only glimmers of improvement surface—the beginning of a smile, the odd chuckle, a moment of serenity. But this hope is quickly dashed when numbness and negativity return. You want your partner and your relationship back, and so you work hard for their recovery. You may hover and check in with them, anxiously looking for clues as to whether they are getting better or worse. It might even get to the point where you are doing so much that it's unhealthy or unhelpful for you and for them.

It may feel as though your loved one's mental health and well-being is your responsibility. They are vulnerable and suffering, and you currently have more resources than they can muster to make sense of all of this and move forward. Your motives may stem from the compassion or empathy you feel for what they are going through.

There are many effective ways to support a partner with depression. Listening and validating, educating oneself about depression and the best treatment options available, and working to increase behavioral activation and change negative thinking are all helpful strategies. But, like Linda, it's not your job to rescue your partner.

You can't change your partner no matter how hard you try. You aren't to blame if they aren't willing or able to change. Change must come from within. In other words, it's your partner—not you—who needs to take the necessary steps to overcome their depression. You can encourage and support, but you can't change them. If you find that you are working harder than your partner is on their recovery, it might be time to step back and reevaluate.

Having Responsibilities Can Help Your Partner

When your partner is depressed, it's tempting to take on all the responsibility around the house—the schedules, the groceries, the finances, the laundry, the yard work. Although this is exhausting for you, it at least ensures that what needs to get done is done. Partners often think that if they just do this one more thing, things will get better. The problem is that the inbox is always full. There will always be more to do. Meanwhile, you are drained and depleted, the situation never changes, and you can't catch up. It's important to recognize that you can't do it all. Even if you could, it may not be the best strategy.

There are times, particularly early in the depression cycle, or during more severe episodes, when you might be doing more than you normally would, to try to help your partner get back on their feet. That might make sense for you provided you feel as though you can see light at the end of the tunnel and your partner is trying to make progress. However, being overinvolved and taking on too much responsibility may be detrimental to you and your partner. Even if you're "all in," it's important to understand that this doesn't mean you do everything. You want to consider what's in your best interest, your partner's, and your relationship's long term. Doing everything for your partner won't help you, because you're likely to burn out, feel resentful, or both.

It's also not helpful for your partner. When you assume all the responsibility, you're unintentionally usurping the control and confidence they would have if they engaged. Clearly, there is a time and a place for taking on more responsibility or holding back. For example, if your partner is experiencing severe and incapacitating depression, you will need to pull more of the weight for a while. Be cautious, however, of making this part of your relationship pattern long term. When being overinvolved becomes part of your pattern, it inadvertently sends a message to the person with depression that they can't do anything. It also sets up an expectation in the relationship that you will ensure that everything is covered. This might result in the opposite of what you intend. It could reinforce your partner to remain stuck in their depression.

Holding back a bit and letting your partner have some responsibility can also be good for them. You may have to be patient and help them reengage gradually, especially at first, but assigning or agreeing on more responsibility bit by bit will give them a sense of accomplishment, which will be reinforcing and likely to help improve their mood. Ask yourself, "Will helping my partner in this way help them or might it negatively impact them? What are the advantages and disadvantages both in the short term and in the long term?" Sometimes doing things for your partner can seem beneficial in the short term but may not be optimal in the long run.

Having Your Own Needs Is Not Selfish

When considering whether you're taking on too much, also ask yourself, "How is helping my partner in this way affecting me?" When you're caught up in the emotional tornado of your partner's depression, it's natural to get into survival mode and focus on the emergency at hand. Your attention shifts to your partner and their well-being, and you can easily neglect to take care of your own needs.

People often feel conflicted about prioritizing their needs. They feel guilty and believe their needs should take a back seat. After all, their loved one is depressed and having a heck of a time just trying to put one foot in front of the other. "How selfish to think that my needs are important right now!"

Taking care of yourself is, however, not selfish. It's also not selfish to want a partner who is present and engaged or to need help and support from them too. In addition, if you don't prioritize your needs, you won't have enough in yourself to support them.

Know Your Limit and Stay within It

"Know your limit and play within it" is a slogan used to help educate people about the risks of gambling and to encourage healthy gaming habits. It's an important lesson for partners of individuals with depression too. Be aware of how your partner's depression is impacting you and do what you can to take care of yourself during this difficult time. There will be times when you need a break or will want to call on others for support. Don't feel guilty about taking care of your needs or be afraid to reach out.

It's so easy to lose yourself in the process. You are coping with a lot. You have lost blood, sweat, and tears fighting the battle for your partner and for your relationship. It's time to recognize that you matter too. Gaining a new perspective, one that doesn't solely define you as a caregiver of a partner with depression, will go a long way toward preserving yourself, focusing on other important relationships, maintaining your well-being, being more hopeful, and improving your relationship.

10

Putting Structure and Routine Back into Your Life

When your partner is depressed, it often feels like every ounce of energy is devoted to picking up the pieces and trying to fit them together into a coherent whole so your partner can improve and you can have some semblance of your relationship back. Supporting a partner with depression is tough and can really test the limits of how much stress, exhaustion, and despair you are able to handle. But life must go on. *Your* life must go on. If your partner doesn't want to join you in meeting up with friends or doing something fun, it's important to do it anyway. You need to have a life outside of caring for your partner.

Aaron was a gym rat. He got up at 5:30 every morning to work out. When a friend at the gym asked how he had managed to care for Bianca for so long and maintain such a positive attitude, Aaron replied, "I'm trying to be my best so I can help my partner. I try to make time to eat right, exercise, meditate, read, and get away with friends. If I didn't do that, we'd both be depressed. I can't afford *not* to take care of myself."

Unlike Aaron, most caregivers of people with depression don't feel equipped to handle the pressure and remain unsure how to manage their own needs. They know that not taking care of their own needs is not what they or their relationship needs, but they don't know how to take care of themself and their partner.

When your partner is depressed, it's easy to feel out of control and stop doing what is healthy and makes you feel good. One way to diminish the impact is to do things you enjoy and have a healthy routine. Otherwise, you can get sucked into a vortex of uncertainty, unpredictability, worry, and tension. The more anxious, stressed, and frustrated you are, the harder it will be to deal with your partner's depression.

It's important to make yourself a priority so that you can get good-quality sleep, exercise, eat well, connect with others, do what you find rewarding, and find time to unwind and relax. This chapter provides guidance on how to do that.

Prioritize Sleep

Jennifer had struggled to get a good night's sleep since Daniel's depression worsened. Daniel would often stay up late watching television or playing video games. Jennifer lay in bed awake each night, worrying about him. When she was finally able to doze off, Daniel would quietly enter the bedroom and unintentionally wake her. She rarely got a full night's rest. In addition to getting a late start each night, her sleep was fragmented because Daniel would toss and turn, disrupting Jennifer's sleep.

The amount and quality of sleep we get significantly impacts both our physical and mental well-being. When we sleep soundly, our bodies work to repair cells, tissues, and muscles, allowing us to recover physically. Consistent, quality sleep enhances performance, improves stamina, and strengthens our immune systems, giving our bodies a better fighting chance against illnesses. Quality sleep also reduces the risk of cardiac problems, such as heart disease and high blood pressure. Furthermore, our mental functioning improves when we get good sleep, sharpening our focus and allowing us to think, concentrate, and remember better. By getting good-quality sleep, we also improve our ability to cope with day-to-day stress.

When sleep is disrupted, because of things such as inconsistent sleep schedules or excessive screen time before bed, our sleep–wake cycle gets out of whack, leading to problems like insomnia. Research demonstrates that poor sleep can negatively impact mental health, increasing the risk of depression, anxiety, and stress.

One way to improve the quality of sleep is to establish healthy habits that promote restorative sleep. These include maintaining a consistent sleep schedule, ensuring your body is ready for bed, and creating an environment that is conducive to sleep.

Set Up a Consistent Sleep Schedule

One of the most effective ways to improve sleep quality is to maintain a regular sleep–wake cycle. This means trying to go to bed and wake up at the same time every day, even on weekends and holidays. This will help regulate your body's internal clock and make your sleep more efficient and uninterrupted, allowing you to feel more refreshed. If you aren't tired, however, it's best to stay up until your head is nodding and then hit the hay. There is a difference between feeling tired and feeling sleepy. If you are already in bed and feeling restless for more than 20 or 30 minutes, get out and do something relaxing until you do feel sleepy and then try again. And don't watch the clock! The best way to experience insomnia is to tell yourself, "Oh my goodness, look at the time. I gotta get to sleep! I only have three hours left until I have to get up!" Having a pad of paper and pen at your bedside and writing down what's keeping you up in the moment can help. Your brain will register that it's on the list and you can let go of the worry until the next day. You might need to engage in this exercise several times a night, and then your sleep will likely improve within a number of days.

There will be times when you end up staying up late because of a social engagement or you just don't feel like going to bed. On those nights when you do stay up longer than usual, the key is to make sure you still wake up at the same time in the morning (no matter how you slept). This will increase your drive for sleep throughout the next day and allow you to sleep better that night. *Sleep drive* refers to your body's increased need for sleep the longer you stay awake. This builds up throughout the day and peaks at night, letting your body know when it's time to rest. Disruptions to sleep drive, like irregular sleep times or naps, can weaken this drive, making it harder to fall asleep at night.

Sleeping in results in what's called *social jet lag*. The body will feel the same way it does when you have taken a flight to another time zone. So, try to get up at the same time every day.

Establish a Relaxing Bedtime Routine

About an hour before bed, start slowing down and engage in activities that are more passive, such as reading, listening to calm music, taking a bath, or practicing relaxation techniques. This signals your body that it's time to wind down and prepare for sleep. Try to avoid things that you find stimulating. And—this is a tough one—put your cell phone and electronics away; for some people, blue light exposure can interfere with the sleep cycle.

Avoiding caffeinated drinks, nicotine, or other stimulants in the late afternoon or evening is also a good idea. These substances can interfere with your sleep. Alcohol is a double-edged sword. Although it can make you feel drowsy initially, it ends up fragmenting your sleep cycles, leading to more frequent awakenings in the night. Minimize your alcohol intake as much as possible. Given all the public media attention to the link between alcohol, cancer, and other negative health outcomes, this will serve you well anyway.

Make Your Environment Work for Sleep

Finally, think about how your bedroom is set up. Most people find they can sleep better if the room is quiet, dark, and cool. You might find earplugs, a white noise machine, or blackout curtains work for you. If you and your partner have different preferences, you might need to agree on what will work for both of you. Although this isn't for everyone, sometimes sleeping in separate beds might be the best solution for a solid night's sleep.

It's important to note that developing good sleep habits, although effective for insomnia, may not be enough. If sleep is a big issue for you, you might consider purchasing a good self-help book, such as *Goodnight Mind* by Drs. Colleen Carney and Rachel Manber. Seeing someone who specializes in cognitive-behavioral therapy for insomnia (CBT-I) may be another good option.

Exercise Regularly

Ironically, when you are steadfast in supporting your partner through their struggles, some of the first things you're likely to sacrifice are the very things that invigorate you. Exercise is one of those activities that can so easily go on the back burner when you're stressed and dealing with so much. Exercise is great not only for physical health; it's also important for your mental health and well-being. Regular exercise can help lift your mood, boost energy, and reduce stress. When we exercise—whether it's a brisk walk or high-intensity training—our bodies release chemicals called *endorphins*, which act as natural mood enhancers. Exercise also helps our bodies regulate other brain chemicals, such as serotonin, which helps improve sleep and mood. If I had a prescription pad, I would prescribe exercise for most clients.

The nice thing about exercise is that you don't have to go all out to reap the benefits. Even a moderate amount of physical activity can have mental health benefits. If you are new to exercise or have mobility issues, start slow and work your way up to what works for you. Go for a walk, stretch, work in some gentle yoga, or do some seated exercises. "Motion is lotion," and even light exercise can enhance mobility, improve joint function, and reduce pain. Your body is meant to move, and when you give it what it needs, it will thank you and pay you back in dividends. It might be wise to check with your physician first to see if there are significant medical issues that would contraindicate an exercise routine.

Whatever amount of exercise you do, the key is to be consistent. Start small and gradually work your way up to what fits with your goals and lifestyle. If you aren't sure where to begin, try doing something that you enjoy, like walking, hiking, swimming, gardening, tai chi, cycling, or dancing. Aim for at least 30 minutes of exercise most days of the week.

If exercise hasn't been part of your schedule for a while, it may take some effort to get going, but it won't take long before it becomes part of your natural routine. Remember that action comes before motivation (see Chapter 5). Don't wait to exercise until you feel motivated; make exercise an important part of your day and you'll find that it won't be so onerous. Once you experience some of the benefits, you'll be more likely to keep at it.

If you're not sure where to start, try an activity you enjoy. Doing something you love increases the chance that you'll stick with it. You don't have to hit the gym either. There are myriad fun and effective ways to get your body moving. Don't let guilt interfere with being active. You need this time to decompress and feel good. It will also give you more gas in the tank to support your partner.

Eat Well

We all know that we should be eating healthier and avoiding highly processed foods. Social media and mass media inundate us with reminders. Ads, articles, and posts flood our feeds with a constant stream of information on the latest diet trend. Although you can choose to pay attention to celebrity endorsements and advice from influencers, maintaining a healthy, balanced diet is simpler than it appears.

Like sleeping and exercise, healthy eating is a cornerstone of physical and mental health. Eating well keeps your energy levels up and bolsters your immune system. And it helps psychologically. For example, the Mediterranean diet is recommended by numerous organizations, including the World Health Organization, the U.S. Centers for Disease Control and Prevention, and the American Heart Association, as a viable way to reduce cardiovascular disease, improve brain health, manage weight, and lessen feelings of anxiety and depression. The Mediterranean diet is rich in omega-3 fatty acids (such as fish), vegetables, fruits, nuts, legumes, whole grains, and healthy fats, like olive oil. These have anti-inflammatory properties, which are associated with reduced stress and negative mood states. This diet is also packed with vitamins, minerals, and antioxidants that support brain health.

A number of things can interfere with eating well. When you're busy supporting your partner, it can be difficult to maintain a balanced diet. This is especially true if your partner has carbohydrate cravings or no appetite at all, a common symptom of depression. Many people with depression turn to comfort foods, like chips, bread, cookies, and cakes, to cope with negative feelings. When this is the case, it's hard to be cognizant of what you eat or maintain a healthy diet. The temptations are ever-present.

The goal is to move toward healthier eating, not strive for perfection. We all cave occasionally and grab an ice-cream cone or bag of Zesty Cheese Doritos (my faves). If you are already eating well, terrific. Keep it up. If you aren't, it may be time to start thinking about what you are putting into your body. A lot of researchers and dieticians are touting the importance of maintaining a healthy gut microbiome (trillions of microbes that play a crucial role in brain health and affect our mood and well-being). In the spirit of moving toward healthier eating, here are a few tips:

- Try to prepare meals and snacks that are dense in nutrients. Fruits, vegetables, lean proteins (like chicken or fish), healthy fats, and whole grains are rich in vitamins, minerals, and antioxidants. We may not crave this, but we tend to feel more energized when snap peas win the battle over chips (snap peas also give us that crunch we often like when snacking).
- Think about preparing meals ahead of time and look at online recipes and cookbooks so you can plan healthy meals for the week.
- Keep healthy snacks around the house. If almonds, yogurt, or fruit are easy to grab, you might be more inclined.
- Do your best to avoid highly processed foods and beverages like sugary snacks and drinks, alcohol, processed meats, refined grains, and ready-to-eat meals. They are associated with heart disease, diabetes, and obesity. They also disrupt gut health and are linked to worse mental health.

Connect with Others

When you're juggling household, childcare, or financial responsibilities along with the multitude of tasks involved in supporting your partner, it might feel as though you don't have time to get out and socialize. Besides, you might feel too exhausted. After a long, emotional day, the thought of getting together with others might be the farthest thing from your mind. Instead, the pull of the couch, a warm blanket, a hot cup of tea, and your favorite series to binge-watch may seem like the best option.

There's nothing wrong with that. Retreating from others and making time for yourself is often a healthy choice. But it may not always be the best choice, especially if solitude becomes a pattern. Getting together with other people, even when you're tired or it seems like more work than it's worth, can help lift your mood, reenergize you, and provide much-needed support. It can also be an opportunity to get active and have fun.

Research clearly demonstrates that having social ties and feeling connected to others is beneficial for our well-being and one of the best ways to live fully. There are also advantages for our physical health. People who have good social connections are not only happier but also tend to live longer. In contrast, feeling lonely and isolated increases the risk of heart disease, depression, and weakened immune systems.

Unfortunately, many of us feel disconnected. In fact, social isolation and loneliness have become such a problem that in January 2018, the U.K. government appointed a Minister of Loneliness. Although this was an important move and one that other countries should consider, what a sad statement of where people are today. A twelve-month investigation into the prevalence of loneliness in the United Kingdom revealed that nine million Brits (14% of the population) suffer from loneliness. The problem hits closer to home too. For example, a 2021 report from Statistics Canada revealed that 1 in 10 Canadians over the age of 15 years report frequently feeling lonely. In 2023, the U.S. Surgeon General's report, *Our Epidemic of Loneliness and Isolation,* suggested that nearly half of U.S. adults are lonely. Now, more than ever, people feel invisible, isolated, and insignificant.

Over the past number of years, I have been on the board of directors for Mental Health Research Canada, an organization that supports stakeholder-driven research that includes people with lived experience in every step of the research. Every few months, since the beginning of the COVID-19 pandemic, we have surveyed Canadians across the country on the state of their mental health (at the time of writing this chapter, we have surveyed over 80,000 individuals). Consistently, across numerous risk factors and indicators, respondents have indicated that social isolation has the greatest negative impact on their mental health.

It takes effort, especially when you're tapped out, but I encourage you to make the effort to connect with others. When you can, opt for in-person interactions over texts or catching up with friends through Facebook, X, or Instagram. Get together with friends and family to have meaningful face-to-face conversations. It's critical for your own well-being and will help provide effective support for your partner.

In addition to the pleasure that connecting with others can bring, reaching out to your friends and family can provide you with emotional support and practical assistance. For example, talking with people can help you process difficult emotions. Your friends and family may also be able to assist with practical things like taking care of your kids so you can have a break or helping with some things on your to-do list.

It's hard to ask for help. You don't want to burden other people, right? They are busy and have stuff going on in their own lives. You aren't off course if you're thinking this way, but you may be applying a double standard. If you had a friend who came to you and said that they were struggling with this, how would you react? I'm guessing you'd want to help them. Your friends are likely to respond similarly.

As noted in Chapter 8, sometimes people are hesitant to get together with others because they feel guilty about leaving their partner at home. During the first five or so years of marriage, Katerina and Luke had a number of good friends and would hang out with them regularly. But then kids came along, things got busy, and, before she knew it, Katerina felt more alone. Although Katerina wanted to get out and socialize, she felt conflicted about leaving Luke alone at home, especially at times when he was really down. Luke would tell Katerina, "Go out. You need to look after you," but Katerina stayed in the house. She rarely got out, except to run errands. To Katerina, getting out of the house and making time for herself meant "abandoning" Luke, and she couldn't bring herself to do it. Having a life and getting together with friends and family is not abandoning your partner. It is a necessity—for your mental and physical health and well-being. It's also important for your partner. Having this time to connect will allow you to recharge, minimize burnout, and be the best support you can be. Try to toss guilt aside and don't sacrifice this important need.

Getting together with others might also be difficult because, when you do, you may feel as though you're always complaining about what's going on in your life. There's always a fire to put out, always a problem. Sela didn't want to meet up with friends because she felt "there's nothing good going on in my life right now. I don't want to just talk about negative stuff. I also don't always want to hear everybody's positive stuff either. On top of that, I don't want others to feel bad about having all these good things going on in their life while nothing good is happening in mine. It's just way easier to not hang out with people." This is a tough scenario because, in some respects, Sela is correct. If the conversation always turns to the negative, it might be difficult for others to interact, which, no doubt, creates a vicious cycle.

In this case, you might want to limit sharing personal struggles with just a few good friends and be aware of how much you air your grievances. Consider balancing this with some activities where you are getting together just to have a good time. For other friends who may not be in your inner circle, you may choose to share less and focus more on healthy distractions. In these instances, try to use your outings to feel refreshed and active and be around others who are fun, positive, and rewarding.

Another reason it may be difficult to get in touch with others is that you're trying to navigate how much to tell others about your loved one's depression. Although respecting your partner's privacy is important, you may decide to open up to a limited number of people, those you can trust will keep your information confidential and be a solid support for you. Be judicious about who you share your personal details with and how much you share. But remember that with vulnerability comes intimacy. You might find that sharing what you are going through can help deepen your relationships. Your friends also can't read your mind. If they don't know what you're going through, they won't be able to help. So, reach out, be honest, ask for support.

Do What You Find Rewarding

Fritz's garage smelled of cedar and sawdust, a strong aroma that always brought a smile to his face. He adored woodworking and would lose himself for hours coming up with new creations. He loved each phase of a new project: the thrill of finding the wood with the perfect grain, the precise cut from the table saw, the smooth glide of the plane, and the finer and finer sandpaper that transformed rough edges into polished perfection. It wasn't just a hobby; it was his passion. But after Liz became depressed, Fritz stopped doing what he loved. The garage, once a sanctuary for him, instead became a place of guilt. In his relentless attempt to be a supportive partner, Fritz had forgotten his own needs.

When your time and energy are focused on supporting your loved one, it's easy to forget or neglect to do what you're passionate about, find stimulating, or enjoy. Your mind may be filled with frenzied thoughts like "I have too much to do," "My partner's needs are more important right now," or "How can I make time for fun activities when my partner is in so much pain?" When you do push to do something for yourself, a nagging internal voice may trigger feelings of guilt.

For several reasons, it's important to do things that you find rewarding even when your partner is depressed. In fact, your partner's depression is arguably all the more reason to do things you like. First, your needs are important to attend to as well. You need to feed your soul, or you will find the monotony and never-ending grind of your routine crushing and suffocating. Second, constantly focusing on your partner's needs to the exclusion of your own can make you emotionally, physically, and mentally exhausted. This can lead to your own mental health problems. Third, when you're running on empty, you'll be less effective at providing support and may even start to resent your partner. Another benefit of engaging in activities you find rewarding is that you can model to your partner the importance of self-care.

After several months, Fritz noticed he was feeling lethargic and blah and decided he needed to do something about it. On his way to the pharmacy to pick up medication for Liz, Fritz popped into the hardware store. There was nothing he was looking for specifically; it just felt good to wander through the familiar aisles. Almost impulsively, he bought a sleek new router (a power tool used to shape wood with precision). Although Fritz hesitated a bit when he returned home, he managed to push through his guilt. "I need to take care of me too!" he thought. He grabbed a walnut plank and turned on the router. For him, the whine of the motor was a comforting sound. He smiled as the router bit carved a clean edge, the wood shavings curling away on the floor.

If you already have hobbies or interests that you enjoy but have discontinued, pursue them again. Try to manage the guilt by telling yourself that this is important not only for you but for your partner and your relationship too. If you aren't an enthusiast for anything specifically, try a few things out and see if they bring you a sense of reward and pleasure. This could be as simple as picking up a crossword puzzle, joining a book club, or committing to regular hikes. It could involve joining a recreational sport. You might consider activities that get you outside—there is something about being out in fresh air that's good for the soul. Be deliberate in coming up with activities that you can do in the warmer months and in the colder months. You could also consider volunteering. Considerable research demonstrates that we feel better when we give than when we receive. Pouring your efforts into something like a charity organization or food bank might be rewarding and provide an opportunity to meet new people who share similar values. If you find it tough to come up with ideas, check out the list in Chapter 5. Doing what you find rewarding will allow you to approach things with more energy and zest. You will also feel as though you have a life beyond caring for your partner.

Make Time to Relax

Another important way to unwind and take care of yourself is to do some relaxation training. Depending on your interests and what fits for you, you have several options. Common to all of them is learning deep breathing.

Deep breathing involves consciously slowing down and deepening your breath. As an experiment, place your hand on your chest and your stomach and see how you breathe. What you want to do is have your stomach move and your chest stay more or less still (when we use our chests, we tend to shallow-breathe, a response consistent with feeling stressed). Instead of sucking air in, try to expand your diaphragm. By expanding your belly, you will automatically draw air in. If you want to see the "experts" do it, watch babies breathe. They use their tummies. Interestingly, as we get older, we tend to unlearn how to breathe diaphragmatically. We stick out our chests and suck in our stomachs, producing the effect that is opposite what we want. Taking slower, deeper breaths can help reduce tension, stress, anxiety, and improve our focus and clarity of thinking.

TRY THIS: DEEP BREATHING

If you want to give it a shot, here's the basic idea behind deep breathing:

1. Inhale deeply through your nose. Allow your lungs to fill with air. You are aiming to expand your belly, not raise your chest.
2. Hold it in for a couple of seconds.
3. Then slowly exhale through your mouth.
4. Continue breathing slowly for a few minutes.

A related strategy is called *box breathing.* Picture a doorframe. On the left, long side of the door, breathe in slowly through your nose. At the top, hold your breath. On the right side, breathe out slowly through your mouth. Finally, hold it for the bottom of the doorframe.

Why a doorframe? I often work with patients who are experiencing anxiety. They can easily think of a door when feeling revved up because they are often looking for the exit to escape the anxiety-provoking situation. However you decide to slow down your breathing, try doing it a few times a day. You might be pleasantly surprised by how well it can help alleviate stress. If you are feeling strapped for time, try doing some diaphragmatic or box breathing when driving or each time you hit a red light in traffic.

Another relaxation technique is called *progressive muscle relaxation.* This involves tensing and then relaxing different muscle groups in your body, one at a time. By doing this, you discover which parts of your body are carrying tension and learn to release it.

TRY THIS: PROGRESSIVE MUSCLE RELAXATION

Here are the basic steps:

1. Find a quiet, comfortable place to sit or lie down. Close your eyes and relax.
2. Spend two or three minutes deep-breathing.
3. Tighten the muscles in different body parts one at a time, hold it for 5–10 seconds, and then slowly release. Don't constrict your muscles so much that you feel pain but enough that you feel some tension:
    a. Begin with the muscles in your feet. Curl your toes.
    b. Tighten your calf muscles by pointing your toes upward.
    c. Tighten your thigh muscles.
    d. Tighten your glutes (butt muscles).
    e. Stiffen stomach muscles.
    f. Tighten your forearms by clenching your fists, hold, then release.
    g. Shrug your shoulders up toward your ears, hold, then relax and let them drop.

h. Gently press your head back, but not too much, hold, then relax.
i. Scrunch up your face by tightening your eyes and mouth, hold, then relax your face (if you have a tight jaw, or temporomandibular joint disorder, omit this step).

Deep breathing and progressive muscle relaxation are commonly used, but there are many other techniques available. For example, some involve bringing awareness to physical sensations in your body to induce a calming effect (called *autogenic training*). There are also relaxation approaches that involve listening to calm music or sounds or imagining relaxing scenes. All these techniques can help reduce stress. If you're interested, you can check out some relaxation apps and see what works best for you. For example, there's Headspace (which provides a range of guided meditations), Calm (which has calming music and breathing exercises), Breathe (which focuses on deep breathing exercises), and MindShift CBT (which uses cognitive-behavioral therapy principles to manage anxiety). Whatever relaxation approach to choose really depends on what you find most relaxing for you.

I hope that this chapter inspired you to start prioritizing yourself. It's easy to put your needs secondary, but you are important to care for too.

PART THREE

Supporting Your Relationship

11

Common Pitfalls and Thorny Issues

This chapter will help you deal with some of the specific challenges that often come up when dealing with a partner's depression.

When Your Partner Seeks Too Much Reassurance

Charlize and Mike met during a group hike. It was a hot, sticky summer afternoon, and the humidity felt like a wet blanket. Mike had joined the local hiking group several years back through a Meetup app. It was Charlize's first time getting acquainted with the group. Her friend had recommended hiking to meet new people and lift her mood. And it certainly did. When she met Mike, the connection was instant and magnetic. As they walked along the trail, Charlize and Mike had a long conversation. Although they were with a group, it felt as though it was just the two of them. It wasn't long before they decided to date.

Mike wasn't like anyone else Charlize had ever met. He was warm, patient, and kind. He made her feel special. Mike was also a conversationalist, which Charlize hadn't experienced in previous romantic encounters. Charlize had struggled with depression on and off since college, but Mike always seemed to understand. He made her feel safe and never judged her when she was in a depressed mood.

After the initial "honeymoon phase" wore off, however, Charlize fell into another depression and became more anxious about the relationship. She started asking Mike, "Do you still love me?" and "Are you mad at me?" When this started, Mike reassured Charlize, "Of course I love you. You mean the world to me." But Charlize doubted herself and the relationship. The frequency and intensity of her questions increased over time. It got to the point where Charlize was checking multiple times a day. Charlize recognized that this was way too much, but she couldn't help herself. It was like having an itch that wouldn't go away no matter how much you scratched. Initially, Mike patiently reassured her that everything was good. But as the demands for reassurance continued, he started to respond in a less tender, even curt, way: "Char, I told you already. Why do you keep asking again and again? I *just* told you I love you." Mike became irritated at the constant need for reassurance, and Charlize could feel him pulling away. This only increased her anxiety and intensified her behavior. The more convinced she became that she was unlovable and that Mike was dissatisfied with the relationship, the more clingy Charlize became. Her questions were endless when she was with Mike. When he was away at work, she texted him repeatedly throughout the day.

Mike felt suffocated and needed some space. Although he wasn't consciously trying to pull away, Mike started working later and stopped initiating hugs. One evening during dinner, Charlize started in with another round of "Do you still love me?" questions. Mike couldn't take it. "I can't keep doing this," he exploded. "No matter how often I tell you that I love you, you don't believe me and it's never enough!"

What Mike and Charlize were dealing with is a common pattern that shows up when one partner experiences depression. Because of their own anxiety and self-doubt, individuals with depression often feel like a burden to their loved one and fear abandonment. As a result, they start to seek reassurance. At the beginning, loved ones provide assurances that they love their partner and will be there for them, but the anxiety continues and so does the need for validation and comfort. If you have experienced this cycle of excessive reassurance seeking, you know that it becomes aggravating over time and puts a strain on the relationship. Nothing you say or do is enough to convince your partner. You might feel angry or hopeless. You don't want to push your partner away, but you need some breathing room, and you're frustrated that they don't seem to believe you. Your constant assurances provide only temporary relief and, within no time, they're back to checking again. It's an easy pattern for couples to fall into and a difficult one to get out of unless you are aware of what's going on.

Individuals with depression often experience negative thoughts about themselves. When these thoughts intensify, they trigger insecurities about what kind of partner they are and the stability of the relationship. They may become hypervigilant to cues that you are withdrawing and start to interpret neutral (or even positive) behaviors as signs that you are unhappy in the relationship. Getting reassurance is highly reinforcing because it quickly alleviates these fears. But it doesn't sink in, and the doubt resurfaces. So they seek reassurance again . . . and again, and you're stuck in a loop.

Providing reassurance doesn't help the person with depression. Instead, they feel powerless in their ability to manage their emotions and become overly dependent. The very behaviors they use to cope with their sadness can unintentionally push others away, creating a feedback loop that reinforces feelings of worthlessness and isolation. So what can you do to break the cycle?

Be Aware of the Pattern

Being aware of how reassurance seeking unfolds in your own relationship is a good initial step. If you are able, it can be helpful to review with your partner what is happening with their thinking when they have the urge to seek reassurance. How long does it last when you comply with this request? Then what happens? Reviewing the process in a calm and gentle manner might help your partner see that reassurance seeking only temporarily alleviates their insecurities because it doesn't help change their underlying beliefs. You might also want to disclose how this pattern impacts you. You might say something like "I don't mean to withdraw, but it's tough to constantly be bombarded with questions about the legitimacy of my love and commitment. I sometimes need a bit of space, but that doesn't mean I am abandoning you." You could also point out that your feelings of frustration, anger, or even resentment just mean that this is something the two of you need to work out. It doesn't mean that you are giving up on the relationship or that you no longer love your partner.

Help Change Thinking

When someone with depression feels insecure about their relationship, these fears often stem from negative thoughts about themself, like "I'm worthless" or "I'm unlovable." These beliefs, in turn, impact how they interpret their partner's behaviors and the dynamics of the relationship. For example, they might think they're a burden to their partner or they don't offer anything valuable to the relationship. Because of these self-deprecating beliefs, they draw the conclusion that your love is waning or that you want to exit the relationship. This mindset also impacts how they interpret your behaviors. For instance, you might just need some time on your own to collect your thoughts. To your partner, however, this may mean you don't want to be around them or that you're questioning the relationship. Helping them challenge these thoughts can be helpful (see Chapter 6). By helping your partner understand how negative thoughts influence their emotions and reassurance-seeking behaviors, your partner might be more motivated to shift them. For example, what's the evidence that you're going to abandon the relationship? Can your partner come to see that it's not either-or (*all-or-nothing thinking*); that you can both be frustrated and irritated with their behavior *and* still love them?

When I was a young child, my mom used to tuck me in at night and say "I love you, like you." Interestingly, although she always said, "I love you," the "I like you" part wasn't always part of that sentence—and for good reason. I wasn't always a well-behaved kid. I may have done things that bugged her or showed disrespect. But "I love you" was always there. All relationships are characterized by disappointments, frustrations, and irritations, and although we may not like our partner all the time, we can choose to always love them. I used the word *choose* deliberately, because *love* is more of a verb, than just a feeling. It is something we deliberately decide to do. Can you also help your partner understand that you may not like them all the time, but that you do love them and will be there for them? It's an important distinction.

By working through these thoughts, you might be able to help your partner understand their dependency and the reasons they are seeking so much reassurance. A discussion of the pros and cons of reassurance seeking might also be beneficial. Doing this can help your partner recognize that reassurance seeking is not a solution to the problem; it's contributing to the problem.

Response Prevention

Response prevention, a cognitive-behavioral technique common for the treatment of obsessive–compulsive disorder (and other anxiety problems), can also be helpful in managing reassurance seeking. Response prevention involves deliberately refraining from engaging in behavior that will only help anxiety in the short term. In this case, it involves having your partner try to refrain from reassurance seeking even when they feel the need. The basic idea is that giving in to these urges will only temporarily help reduce anxiety and uncertainty about the relationship. By breaking the habit of checking every time they feel discomfort, your partner will learn to tolerate these feelings without relying on reassurance. Although it's not easy, this will help stop the unhelpful cycle.

Although providing assurances to your partner may be well intentioned, it only reinforces the idea that your partner needs reassurance to feel okay.

Instead of checking out the evidence for themselves, they will start to depend on you to gauge whether the relationship is okay. Here are some tips for doing response prevention with your partner:

1. ***Express your concerns and observations.*** Have a conversation with your partner about the pattern you're noticing. You might say, "I've noticed that when you're feeling down you seem to doubt my love and commitment and ask for a lot of reassurance. I keep telling you that I love you and care deeply about you. I don't think this is helping because, over time, you're asking more and more. I want to support you, but I'm concerned that providing reassurance isn't helping either of us. I'm wondering if we could try a different approach?" During this conversation you could help your partner understand how reassurance seeking becomes reinforcing and only temporarily helps their anxiety. Express that you want to help them feel secure over the long haul. This will help your partner see that what you're proposing, although challenging, will better help ease their worries of abandonment and rejection.

2. ***Develop a plan together.*** Try to agree on a plan with your partner. "I love you and I am here to support you, but I need you to know that for *yourself,* rather than regularly checking in with me to see if it's still true. I'm going to try to refrain from answering questions like 'Are you mad at me?' or 'Do you love me?' or 'Do you think I am a burden?' And I need you to try to cut down how often you ask them." You could then ask your partner what they think, and revise the plan. Instead of going cold turkey, for example, you might agree to start by providing reassurance up to three times a day and then reduce this after a few days or a week. You could also chat about what your partner could do to deal with their uncertainty, like writing down their thoughts and examining the evidence. Many couples will say "I love you" before going to sleep or leaving the house in the morning. These could be added to the routine.

3. ***Implement the plan and be consistent.*** Your partner's assignment is to try to refrain from seeking reassurance. Your assignment is to stop (or reduce) giving it. If your partner asks for reassurance, you could remind them about what you've talked about and how this will help them feel more secure if they keep at it. They may feel considerable anxiety with this task, but remember you are helping them deal with these emotions without requiring validation from you. See if they can sit with the anxiety for a bit and ride it out. You may need to start out gradually, but when your partner is no longer asking for reassurance and you aren't providing it, they will learn to tolerate these uncertain feelings, and it will soon pay off for both of you.

4. ***Provide support with response prevention.*** Research demonstrates that response prevention can be more effective when it's combined with support. You aren't simply ignoring your partner's requests, however. Providing reassurance fuels the pattern, whereas providing support promotes adaptive coping. While you are refraining from providing reassurance, it can be helpful to give supportive comments to your partner. When they ask for reassurance, you could mention, "I can't answer that. I can see this is difficult for you. But you know why I'm not answering this question. Deep down, you know how I feel about you. You can get through this." By doing this, you're supporting this new change in behavior without getting caught up in the pattern again. Your partner's emotional needs are valid; it's just that reassurance seeking isn't the best way to meet them. The goal isn't to extinguish dependency entirely—we all need to feel and express love—it's to help your partner do this in a way that is healthy for both of you and the relationship. Response prevention can also be used for other types of reassurance seeking, like asking you whether other people like them or whether they will be okay in a certain social situation. The principle is the same.

It's also important to deliberately reinforce your partner when they are making strides toward reducing reassurance seeking. Let them know you're proud of them for handling their uncertainties the way they did. This can help them keep at it and increase their confidence.

When Your Partner Pushes You Away

In contrast to being highly dependent and seeking reassurance, you might find that your partner tends to push you away, even when you're just trying to help. This can feel confusing, hurtful, and frustrating. You might be working hard to offer support, love, and care to your partner and, rather than appreciating your efforts or inching closer to you, your partner makes you feel rejected and unwanted. It's always the ones we are closest to that end up hurting us the most, right?

There are many reasons your partner may be pushing you away. Depression is often associated with negative thoughts and emotions, like guilt, shame, and hopelessness, which contribute to withdrawing from close relationships. Similarly, your partner may push you away because they may not feel worthy of your love and care and, when you show it, they retreat because they believe they don't deserve it.

Your partner may also feel overwhelmed and unable to engage.

Depression often makes people feel as though even small tasks or interactions are exhausting. Tracy, for instance, tried to offer support and affection to Neo and encouraged him to talk about how he was feeling. However, Neo felt put on the spot and overburdened and reacted by retreating. "I'm fine," he exclaimed. "I don't want to talk about it." Even though Tracy's initiative was coming from a place of love, Neo didn't have the energy or emotional capacity to deal with this conversation and ended up lashing out.

Your partner might also be frustrated with themself that they are a burden on you. They might feel ashamed or guilty about getting support from you. Even though they desperately want and need your help, they end up pushing you away so that they can feel more in control. They may seem self-sufficient, but this is often a guise to protect them from feeling like a burden or from being hurt or rejected.

Sometimes your partner might be pushing you away because they just feel the need to reside in a cocoon and shut the world out. It's not about you; it's the depression that makes it harder to engage with others. Even if they love you and want to connect with you, they get sucked into a pattern of withdrawing and avoiding.

Another reason people with depression often push others away has to do with feeling criticized or misunderstood. The negative mindset so prevalent in depression often results in interpreting even well-meaning comments as criticism. Your partner might be pushing you away because they don't feel understood or validated (see Chapter 2).

When your partner criticizes you or pushes you away, try not to take it personally. Work, instead, to recognize that depression might be clouding how they are viewing the relationship and the love and support you're offering. What your partner expresses may be more a reflection of their emotional pain than how they really feel about you. Understand that your partner's ability to respond or engage with you might vary from day to day. It's difficult to be patient and compassionate when they push you away but try to find and celebrate the wins and regroup with the losses.

Having said that, setting boundaries is also important. Trying to support someone who rejects your help and pushes you away can be frustrating and draining. Individuals with depression often end up unintentionally creating the very stress that contributes to their depression, due to difficulties managing their emotions, repetitive negative thinking, perfectionism, excessive standards for themselves, and avoidance. They don't mean to create stress, but they end up making life more stressful for themselves and others because of how they are managing their thoughts and emotions.

Your partner may feel agitated and irritable and lash out with anger or insults. This makes sense given how they are feeling, but that doesn't make it acceptable. In these circumstances it's important to know how much you're willing to take and when the line is crossed. In some instances you may want to call out your partner when they make hurtful comments or push you away: "I know you're struggling, but I need to be spoken to with more respect. We are partners and need to treat each other with love and care." If the behavior continues, you may want to let your partner know that you're going to leave the situation for a bit so that you can both cool off. The behavior your partner shows to you may be colored by their depression, but that doesn't make it easy or acceptable. Try to respond in a way that is calm and matter-of-fact and be clear about how you want to be treated. You matter too.

You Might Be Enabling Your Partner's Depression

Another difficult dynamic to navigate when your partner is depressed is how much to help and support them and when this becomes too much. Shelly constantly tried to take the higher road and "fight the good fight" when it came to supporting her husband, Dwayne. She was always there for Dwayne, making sure he was okay and rarely leaving the house for fear that he might feel abandoned. Shelly was constantly making meals for Dwayne, getting him a hot cup of tea, and checking in on how he was doing. It got to the point where supporting Dwayne almost became part of Shelly's personality. Caring for Dwayne was her primary focus and became an important part of her self-identity. What Shelly didn't realize, however, was that the more she did for Dwayne, the less he did for himself. Shelly felt exhausted, and Dwayne became more helpless.

Sometimes you might unintentionally keep your partner stuck by working so hard to help. Ola understood all too well the dynamic of doing too much for her partner, Mohamed. She could hardly help herself. Ever since Mohamed became depressed, Ola would try to meet his every need, whether he expressed it or not. Over time Mohamed became more reclusive and dependent. Rather than getting better, he seemed to be deteriorating. It got to the point where Ola thought, "He can't do anything for himself anymore."

Ola then tried a different strategy. She wanted to support Mohamed but realized that her constant help in every situation was hindering him from doing things for himself, usurping his self-confidence, and maintaining his hopelessness and helplessness. When Mohamed asked Ola to pick something up for him from the store, Ola would respond, "Okay, but why don't you come with me?" At first Mohamed refused and Ola would pick up the item anyway, but over time she realized that Mohamed wanted to do things and then felt bad that he couldn't. She started to encourage Mohamed to do more, bit by bit. Although it was difficult to stick to the plan consistently, encouraging Mohamed to take on more responsibilities helped him regain his confidence.

Take a moment to think about how your behavior might be impacting your partner's depression. Do you fall into the trap of doing too much for them? Are there things you can change so that they might gain more energy and confidence? If you are going to try to tip the scales in favor of helping your partner do more, start small and build slowly from there. You might even let your partner in on what you are trying to accomplish by doing this or come up with a plan together. Be consistent but not rigid. There are times when it's important to lend a hand and support. Keep in mind what's best for your partner (and for you) not only in the moment but also in the long term.

Another common way loved ones try to help their partner is by becoming overprotective. For instance, you might help your partner avoid social contact by allowing them to stay home and making excuses for their absence. When this happens, you risk isolating your partner or causing them to become too dependent on you. Alternatively, you might be inclined to ensure that you are by your partner's side whenever the two of you are out. Although the intention is good (you want your partner to feel comfortable), the outcome often is not.

Rob joined Tanya everywhere they went. He would never wander off at the grocery store or the mall because he knew that Tanya was anxious that she might have a panic attack. So he was with her in every aisle and walked beside Tanya along every hallway. This comforted Tanya and made her feel more at ease, but she never learned that she could handle being apart while shopping. She became more dependent on Rob, which didn't help either of them. She felt clingy and dependent, and Rob felt like he had no autonomy. Eventually the couple decided to work on this. They agreed that Rob would be in the next aisle for a period of just three minutes at first. Then they extended the time to five minutes, and Rob would wander away one aisle farther. Eventually, Tanya was able to do some shopping on her own. She felt better about herself and less reliant on Rob as an emotional crutch.

When Sexual Intimacy Ain't What It Used to Be

Another difficulty you may be dealing with involves the lack of physical intimacy with your partner. Sexual intimacy is often seen as an important part of a relationship, contributing to satisfaction, connection, happiness, and communication. Whether sexual intimacy is essential to a relationship, however, depends on the specific couple. Sexuality is one way of demonstrating love and affection for your partner, but other ways of expressing and experiencing intimacy, like trust and emotional support, are equally or more important.

Problems with sexual intimacy can arise at any time in any relationship. When one member of a couple is experiencing depression, however, difficulties with sexual intimacy are even more common and can put a lot of strain on a relationship. There are often feelings of frustration and hopelessness and fears you are drifting farther apart as a couple.

There are a variety of reasons sexual intimacy can be challenging in this situation. Individuals with depression often find it difficult to feel interested in things that used to bring them pleasure (a symptom called *anhedonia*), including sex. Other common symptoms of depression include low energy and impaired motivation. When your partner is feeling lethargic and chronically exhausted, it's difficult to muster the desire or ability to have sex. Although depression often impacts sexual desire and functioning, it is important not to blame your partner but to consider other factors. For example, if you are being critical of your partner or acting aggressively, they are less likely to be "in the mood."

For many people, especially women, having sex is also tied to emotional closeness. When someone is depressed, they may shut down emotionally because they feel irritable or emotionally numb. This can impact both the individual with depression and their partner. For example, when Anna's partner, Scott, was going through depression, he started to shut down emotionally. He couldn't open up about what was going on with him, which left Anna feeling emotionally distant. Even though they continued to have sex periodically, it felt disconnected, as though sex was no longer tied to intimacy. As a result, Anna started to lose interest.

If you are feeling pushed away or getting signals that your partner isn't interested in sex, or they aren't as emotionally expressive as they used to be, it's tough to keep initiating and pursuing them. You may eventually give up, feeling like you can only be "rejected" so much. You might take it personally, thinking that your partner is no longer interested in you or that your physical attractiveness has faded away. This can lead to a cyclical pattern that makes things worse.

It's also possible that your partner doesn't seem interested in sex because of the beliefs they have about themself. For instance, it is common for people with depression to feel inadequate or worthless. They may also feel unattractive or question how much their partner loves them. It's hard to imagine being loved when you feel so hollow and insignificant. And it's tough to conjure up sexual prowess when you aren't feeling good about who you are or experience guilt or shame about being a burden.

When depression impacts someone's sexual drive, it can also lead to performance anxiety. For example, an individual might worry that they won't be able to have an erection or achieve orgasm. This anxiety can, in turn, interfere with their performance. On the other hand, someone might not be able to become lubricated and worry that their partner will interpret this as though they aren't interested, which can also lead to avoiding sexual advances.

Another possibility is that your partner is experiencing some form of sexual dysfunction. Studies indicate that approximately 63% of men and 83% of women with major depressive disorder experience some form of sexual dysfunction. These figures are much higher than in the general population, where 34% of men and 41% of women report having a current sexual problem.

Most individuals with depression have diminished sex drive. In addition, most antidepressants have side effects that can cause sexual dysfunction. This can include reduced sex drive, difficulty reaching orgasm, problems getting or maintaining an erection, and vaginal dryness or discomfort, which can make intercourse uncomfortable or even painful. Although common, the side effects from antidepressants won't impact everyone's sexual functioning. In fact, in many cases antidepressants can help restore one's sex drive because their mood improves and they feel better.

As you can see, the reasons for sexual difficulties vary widely. If you and your partner are having difficulty with sexual intimacy, you might consider the following steps. Before we get into that, however, I want to point out one caveat. Pardon the pun, but sex can be a touchy subject. Much of the research on sexuality comes from Western cultural beliefs. For example, the ideas that sex is about mutual satisfaction and that an important goal is to communicate openly about your relationship are not true for every culture. With that caution in mind, here are some things to try, assuming that they fit with your personal and cultural background.

1. ***Try to have a realistic perspective and avoid comparing your sex life to* Fifty Shades of Grey.** People rarely talk with family and friends about their sex life. Consequently, it can be difficult to have a realistic understanding of "normal" sexual functioning and it's easy to compare yourself to idealistic standards, often portrayed in movies or pornography. Each person's experience is unique, and we can often hold on to misconceptions like "Our sexual

desire should be in sync" or "If I am attracted to my partner, I should be physically aroused." These standards are biased.

2. ***For now, don't expect your partner to have the same interest in sex as they used to.*** Be patient and realistic about what they can or cannot do during this time. It may take some time before your sex life returns to normal.

3. ***Try to focus on the relationship itself.*** If you work to communicate effectively, demonstrate support, and minimize judgment (of yourself or your partner), you will be more likely to create an environment that is conducive to a more active sex life.

4. ***Work on trying to understand what factors might be impairing sexual intimacy.*** Could it be that the two of you haven't been communicating as well as you could? Does there need to be more romance? It's easy to attribute the problem to your partner or their depression. Avoid blaming each other.

5. ***Let your partner know that you miss the physical closeness.*** If sex is off the table for now, try to work on sharing other forms of intimacy like cuddling, hugging, or massage if your partner is okay with this. Try to cuddle and touch without the expectation that this will lead to sex. You might have to state this clearly and stick to it, unless they initiate.

6. ***Avoid personalizing.*** When you take it personally, you will be more likely to stop initiating, may become resentful, or could lose interest in sex yourself. It's hard to continue if your partner is always rejecting your attempts to initiate sex. The difficulties aren't a reflection of you or your attractiveness. They stem from the complications surrounding depression. If you find that you are doing this, it might be helpful to deal with your own thoughts and reactions. For example, if you feel as though your partner's lack of interest in sex means that they don't love you, try to examine the evidence for these thoughts and look for alternative explanations. Could it be because they are tired or overwhelmed with stress, or could this be a side effect of medication? Remember that a thought is a hypothesis, not a fact (see Chapter 6).

7. ***Communicate openly with your partner.*** Sex is a topic that couples often find difficult to discuss. Mia and Ian were together for nearly 10 years. For the last five years, their sex life was unsatisfying to Mia. She would always be the one to initiate and, when she did, Ian would pleasure her orally or through manual stimulation but no longer seemed interested in intercourse. Ian had difficulty maintaining an erection and felt embarrassed that he wasn't as virile as he used to be. Every time Mia would attempt to touch Ian's genitals, he would gently push her hand away. Mia eventually built up the courage to

speak with Ian and the couple found solutions that worked for both. As mentioned earlier, there are cultural differences in sexual experiences, expectations, and communication so an open discussion is not for everyone. However, when there is persistent disinterest or sexual dysfunctions that are interfering with making love, silence can create loss of intimacy. Don't pretend there isn't a problem. In most cases, this will only make things worse.

8. ***If sexual intimacy is compromised because of a sexual dysfunction or the side effect of medication, have your partner speak with their physician.*** They can come up with alternatives and solutions that may work. It's common to feel shy having this discussion, but family doctors have heard it all. Nothing your partner says will surprise them, and not dealing with it won't be helpful in the long run.

9. ***Consider seeing a sex therapist.*** There are several strategies that will foster better communication and help you regain sexual intimacy. For example, sex therapists sometimes work with clients on a procedure called *sensate focus*. This exercise involves having the couple refrain from intercourse and orgasm for a period and focus instead on sensual touch. The goal is just to experience pleasure and reduce the pressure to perform. Eventually, once the pressure subsides, couples can slowly move toward intercourse.

10. ***Finally, don't feel guilty for wanting to have sex.*** It's perfectly natural to want to experience sexual intimacy with your partner.

The Shift in Dynamics when Your Partner Improves

If your partner has started to improve, the bond between you also may have improved. Your tone with each other may be lightened and your interactions less negative. If that represents your journey, great. This isn't the case for everyone.

This might come as a surprise—especially after you have been working so hard to help your partner improve and wishing so desperately for this day to come—but you might have mixed feelings when your partner starts to feel better. On one hand, you are happy to see them improve and feel the burden lift from both of you. But with improvement comes change and change, even positive change, takes some getting used to. To this point, your relationship may have been defined largely by your partner's depression and your role as caregiver. Their improvement might be confusing to you and might shift the balance of power in the relationship. A considerable amount of your time and energy has been devoted to supporting your partner and helping them feel better. Now that you aren't "needed" as much for support, you might feel a little lost and wonder what your role in the relationship is now.

When your partner improves, they will also become more engaged and start to socialize again. Maybe they are interested in reconnecting with you both emotionally and sexually. This change, however, might be difficult to adjust to. You may not quite feel ready for this. Perhaps you are harboring resentment for the way things have been or built up some emotional walls. There may be some anger that you need to work through. Allow yourself to be honest about what you went through during the depression and let your partner know that you need this validation. It was tough on you. It was rough on your relationship. Be patient with each other and try to rebuild your emotional connection gradually. You might also wonder if this is a temporary, short-lived improvement and be bracing yourself for the next low. It can take some time to adjust to these changes and rebuild the relationship.

Another change that often takes place is the dynamic in the relationship. During the depression, you may have risen to the occasion and taken on more of the responsibilities for the house, finances, kids, and relationship. You were the organized one. You were the stronger one. Now that your partner is improving, the balance of power may be reconfigured. Your partner may have shifted from being at a place of helplessness and dependence to feeling stronger and more capable. This is another dynamic that may take time to adjust to.

When you are both ready, check in with each other, recognize the shifting dynamics, and talk it through. The focus of your conversations will likely change. You might move from discussing your partner's symptoms and how they are doing to how you can reconnect now that the dust has settled. Discuss with your partner how the roles changed during the depression and how you can renegotiate them now. It may take a bit of open discussion and trial and error, but try to experiment with how roles and responsibilities can be more balanced.

Depression and Relationship Distress Go Hand in Hand

Many people who have partners with depression report feeling burdened. Interactions are often negative and characterized by blame and hopelessness. Communication difficulties seem to pervade all conversations, and it feels like the problems keep mounting with no resolution in sight. Being with someone who is depressed can be draining and negatively impact your own mental health. Every comment from your partner may seem derogatory toward themself and you. This is hard to cope with.

How you manage this experience, however, can make a big difference in helping or hindering your partner's depression and your relationship. Not surprisingly, individuals who adapt and adjust to the changes they see in their partner fare better than those who feel overwhelmed. When people can't seem to cope with their partner's depression, they tend to withdraw their support, feel less connected, and experience more conflict.

Relationship distress can also impact your partner's depression. When your partner perceives less support, or that your interactions are filled with criticism and hurt, they are more likely to pull away further or do the opposite—seek reassurance and support. However, because they aren't at their best, they may not communicate positively or demonstrate gratitude for all your efforts. This impacts how you feel and respond. You might feel underappreciated or be unsatisfied and lessen your support over time. After a while, you might be blaming each other for how you are feeling.

The good news is that, by recognizing that a reciprocal relationship exists between depression and relationship distress, you might both be in a better position to figure out how to intervene. Helping your partner feel better *and* reducing relationship distress will likely have a positive impact on both. By using the strategies in this book, you will be able to look for solutions and work together to change some of the dynamics in your relationship. The next three chapters provide strategies for managing your relationship by thinking differently about your partner, effectively communicating and problem solving, and learning how to accept some of those aspects of the relationship that are difficult, if not impossible, to change.

12

The Power of Negative Thinking

Samantha and Jack have been married for 15 years. The beginning of their relationship was characterized by mutual respect, admiration, and love. They felt they were each other's soul mate, sharing interests, sense of humor, goals, and values. They genuinely enjoyed each other's company and were rarely apart, except during work hours. They felt remarkably grateful for each other and were acutely aware of how the relationship enriched their respective lives. Their friends and family often joked about how their honeymoon never seemed to end.

Samantha and Jack also never seemed to argue. If one of them did something that wasn't thoughtful or rubbed their partner the wrong way, it slipped away like Teflon. It wasn't viewed as malicious, selfish, or intentional. When Jack showed up late without telling Samantha that he got held up at work, for example, Samantha gave him the benefit of the doubt and attributed the cause to some benign factor: "He must have a lot on his plate if he forgot to let me know." Conversely, positive things stuck like Velcro. It was as though Samantha and Jack each wore rose-colored glasses.

Things changed when Jack fell into a deep depression and started to withdraw from everyone, including Samantha. This hurt Samantha deeply, but at first she was fully supportive of Jack. She did everything in her power to help him feel better. But as the pattern of withdrawal and avoidance lasted longer and longer, it was more difficult for Samantha to feel connected the way she used to, and she began to pull away from Jack. Her thinking also changed. Instead of seeing and valuing Jack's positive qualities, Samantha started to dwell on his shortcomings. When Jack forgot to pick the kids up from school, Samantha concluded that he was lazy rather than having the understanding thoughts she used to have. Samantha started to see Jack's behaviors in a more negative light, as though her perception of Jack reversed completely. Now the positive things glided off like Teflon and the negative clung like Velcro.

Often, when we are in long-term relationships, thoughts about our partners can veer off track. Sometimes the very characteristics that attracted you to your partner fade in their luster or become the things you now detest. Over time, your partner's kind-heartedness can look more like self-sacrifice. The confidence you may have been attracted to is now seen as arrogance and self-absorption. What you used to see as a fun, laid-back personality now gets viewed as avoidance of responsibility and an inability to take anything seriously. Spontaneity morphs into unreliability. It's painful when early admiration for your partner transforms into disillusionment. Add partner depression to the mix, and negative thoughts can intensify quickly. When dealing with a mountain of stress, turmoil, and despair, it can be difficult to see redeeming qualities in your partner or your relationship.

Understanding how negative thinking about your partner develops and is maintained will put you in a better position to know how to turn it around. The goal isn't necessarily to return to rose-colored relationship glasses, but to at least change the lenses to see your partner less negatively. By applying strategies to help you change your thinking, you will be able to put on "corrective lenses" that allow you to see your partner with 20/20 vision. This new vantage point will, in turn, help you deal with future interactions in a calm, objective way that can help break the cycle of negativity. You will also feel better, and your partner's behavior may change as well.

Partner Schemas and Relationship Lenses

As humans, we naturally categorize and organize information so that we can process it more efficiently. When we learn something new, it takes a lot of time, energy, and resources to grasp the material and become proficient. In Chapter 6, you reflected on when you learned to drive a car and how it took substantial concentration and effort at the beginning. But it didn't take long before you were driving without much thought and quickly able to focus on other things, like the music you were listening to or the conversation you were having with your fellow passenger. All the motor skills involved in driving—from steering to braking—became automated. Our brains develop schemas for what we learn so that we know what to expect and can carry out tasks without taking up too much brain power.

A schema is like a mental framework that we use to understand and organize information. Our brains make sense of the world by grouping things that are similar, recognizing patterns, developing scripts, and predicting what to expect. When you walk into a restaurant, for example, your mind already has a script ready that makes the process run smoothly. You know that you'll be seated and choose something from the menu. You are prepared for a waiter to come to your table and ask what you would like to order. And (although you may be taken aback by the cost) you aren't surprised that you are presented with a bill and are expected to pay for the meal.

When we learn something new, it takes time to get the hang of it and process the information. When you started your job, for example, you were likely uncertain and maybe a bit discombobulated. You might have felt like it would take forever to learn everything to be comfortable in your new environment and meet expectations. Have you ever seen a new employee at a cash register in a grocery store or retail shop? They are easy to spot. As you have likely experienced, they are much slower than other clerks to ring up the items for purchase. Sometimes they need to call another employee over for assistance because they haven't yet developed a mental blueprint (or schema) for their job. With time, however, they can deal with all the nuances of the job with ease, because their experience gets stored in memory and becomes familiar.

Schemas are kind of like the brain's way of filing information, similar to having folders on your computer that hold data. Just like you might create different folders for work, financial information, and personal stuff, we develop schemas for different things like how we understand ourselves, friends, and partners. When we encounter new information, our brains try to determine which folder it should be filed in. If we don't have a folder for this information yet, our brains create a new one. Over time, experiences and memories get placed into different folders. If they are similar, they get filed in the same folder. The more files we have of related information, the easier and faster it is to understand incoming information that fits our preexisting beliefs and expectations.

When Schemas Hurt Rather than Help

Schemas are helpful because they allow us to process information faster, predict what might happen in different situations, and respond automatically in familiar circumstances. When information doesn't quite fit our beliefs and expectations, we tend to either ignore it or adjust our schemas and create a new folder that fits this information. Although schemas can help us quickly process information, there are times when they can be problematic.

Sometimes we can develop schemas about ourselves or others that are biased. An obvious example is when we use mental shortcuts to stereotype others. When using stereotypes about underrepresented or racialized groups, for example, we overgeneralize and reduce individuals to a single identity or trait, which can lead to discrimination or other negative consequences.

Schemas can also be harmful in the case of depression. People with depression often exhibit negative *self*-schemas. Because of this, negative thoughts and information get filtered into their "folders" without questioning whether they are true. And the opposite happens with positive situations. When something bad happens, someone with depression is likely to think that it is their fault (it's internal), will last a long time (it's stable), and applies to everything (it's global). They didn't get the job they applied for, and they jump to attributions of "I'm not good enough" (internal), "I always mess up" (stable), and "I won't succeed at anything" (global).

At the same time, individuals with depression tend to minimize or disqualify positive experiences (see Chapter 6). Someone compliments them on the great job they did on a presentation and their minds go to "They are probably just saying that to be nice" (external), "I was lucky that I had a kind audience" (unstable), and "It wasn't rocket science—it was only because the topic was easy to cover" (specific). I was working with a client recently who received a national award for a company she worked for. This person was convinced that she got the award because the company knew she was struggling and gave it to her out of pity. It took a lot to help her see that she deserved this recognition and that it was grounded in hard work and excellence, not sympathy.

The schemas we develop for our partners can also become skewed and twisted over time. If you have a positive schema of your partner (as Samantha and Jack did at the beginning of their relationship), you are more likely to interpret their behavior in a positive (or at least neutral) way. Let's say you left a voicemail or text for your partner, and they didn't respond for a while. If you had a positive schema (or rose-colored glasses) in which you viewed your partner as generally caring, thoughtful and supportive, you might think, *They were probably just busy. They'll respond as soon as they can.* On the other hand, if your partner schema was negative, you'd be more likely to view their behaviors unconstructively, thinking, *They're ignoring me and don't care what I have to say. I'm not a priority to them.* Over time, the negative information continues to get copied and pasted into our partner folder and their positive behaviors don't register. They are filtered out—they don't get saved, or they end up in the brain's trash folder.

How Schemas Create Expectations of Our Partners

Just as we develop a script for what to expect when we go to a restaurant, we also develop scripts of what we expect of our partners. With a negative partner schema, the positive characteristics and attributes of our partner become like Teflon and the negative characteristics stick like Velcro. The more we view our partner's behaviors in a less forgiving way, the more our folders fill up with negative information.

In addition to influencing how you interpret your partner's behaviors, partner schemas also impact what you pay attention to. For example, if your relationship glasses are less than rosy, you'll be more likely to pay attention to negative things your partner does and fail to notice the positive things.

A fascinating experiment was run in the late 1990s that examined how our attention can be focused so intently on certain things that we miss the obvious. The experiment involved showing a short video of two groups of three players, half wearing white shirts and half wearing black shirts. The players moved around and passed a basketball to each other. The instructions for the study participant were simple: "Count how many times the players wearing white pass the basketball." Partway through the video, a person dressed in a gorilla costume walks in between the players for five seconds. They even stop midway and beat their chest. You'd think this would be obvious and catch your attention, right? Well, no. About 50% of the research participants missed seeing the gorilla entirely! If you want to test this out with some friends who aren't aware of the experiment, check out the YouTube video *www.theinvisiblegorilla.com.*

Imagine missing something so obvious! We do it all the time. We often miss things that are right in front of us because our attention is directed elsewhere. We also tend to focus our attention on things we expect to see. It's almost as though we are wearing psychological blinders. If you have ever ridden a horse or taken a carriage ride through a city, you will have seen blinders—small pieces of leather (or plastic) attached to a horse's bridle, positioned next to their eyes. The purpose of blinders is to block the horse's peripheral vision to minimize distractions and keep the horse focused on the path ahead. Metaphorically, we can sometimes wear psychological blinders when we selectively pay attention to the negative things our partner does and fail to see, or ignore, the positive things.

Remember earlier when we discussed how our brains are wired to categorize and organize information? How we create these mental folders? We pay more attention to what we expect to see because of these schemas or relationship glasses. When we expect to see something, our brains make it easier for that information to slide (almost mindlessly) into our mental folders. Meanwhile, stuff that doesn't fit with our preexisting beliefs is often ignored, disqualified, or discarded. In other words, we don't just see what's there; we see what we expect to see.

Think about this in the context of your relationship. Are you wearing tinted glasses that are impacting how you view your partner? If that's the case, you will be more likely to notice things that are congruent with your negative partner schema and less likely to detect information that doesn't fit. Our memories work the same way. When feeling negative about our partner, we tend to conjure up related memories and images. So, when our relationship glasses get less rosy and more tinted, this impacts how we view, remember, and process information about our partners. We pay attention to their faults and miss seeing their strengths. We think about the times they upset us or let us down rather than remembering the times they supported us and made us feel special. We interpret their behavior in a negative rather than positive light. This, in turn, makes our partner schemas even stronger—negative information gets filed into the mental folder and positive information gets dumped into the trash folder.

How Negative Schemas Multiply

The metaphor of partner schemas being like relationship glasses or mental folders isn't optimal, however, because it doesn't account for the fact that these thoughts are all interconnected. It would be more accurate, I suppose, to view the folder as a large room with all the files overlapping across the floor. Because of how connected each file is, lighting a match to one of the files would make fire spread quickly across the entire floor. When we have a negative partner schema, the activation of one belief is likely to cascade to others. Let's say that your partner forgot to call their doctor to make an appointment or left their dirty shoes on the carpet. Although frustrating, that behavior probably isn't enough to rile you up too much. But when negative thoughts and memories of your partner are interconnected, one negative behavior isn't seen as an isolated event. Instead, thoughts go to other times when they have let you down or disappointed you.

Samantha arrived home from work, said hi to Jack, dropped her purse off by the door, hung up the car keys, and changed into sweats and a T-shirt. As she was starting to get supper ready, Samantha noticed that the dishwasher hadn't been emptied even though Jack promised to do it earlier that morning. She called out to Jack, "I thought you said you would empty the dishwasher!?"

"Oh, shoot. I meant to do that," Jack replied. Samantha's frustration brewed as her mind flooded with recent memories: "Last week, he was going to pick up his prescription but forgot and I had to do it. We used to share the cooking and cleaning; now Jack just doomscrolls on his phone. He left his laundry on the floor after I had cleaned up the bedroom. He made a sarcastic comment about me in front of our friends when we were out for dinner. Ugh, can he do anything right?" She blurted out, "You always say you're going to do something and never follow through!" Her reaction stemmed not from this one incident, but from the negative thoughts and memories that had been piling up in her mental folder. These interconnected files led Samantha to believe that she was invisible, that her needs didn't matter, and that she was alone in the relationship.

Strategies for Shifting Your Partner Schemas

Fortunately, there are strategies that can help you shift your partner schemas and modify your relationship lenses. These strategies involve learning to:

1. Notice a negative shift in your emotions and pay attention to what they are telling you.
2. Change your thinking about your partner so that it is accurate and not biased by negative partner schemas or relationship glasses.
3. Remember the qualities that initially attracted you to your partner.
4. Train yourself to notice your partner's positive behaviors (and reinforce these).

Use Negative Feelings as a Signal (Not a Conclusion)

If you think about it, you'll realize negative feelings are not harmful in and of themselves. They are just feelings. They may be intense and difficult to control, but they are merely feelings, neither good nor bad. It's what you do with your emotions that can be positive or negative. For example, just because you feel a negative emotion doesn't mean it's inevitable that you lash out or give your partner the silent treatment. There may be other alternatives to managing this feeling.

It can be helpful to view negative emotions as a signal—a signal that something needs to change. Physical pain, for example, lets us know that we need to do something to prevent further damage to our skin, muscles, joints, or tendons. Experiencing acute pain from touching a hot stove signals that you need to quickly remove your hand from a hot element to protect yourself. Likewise, the emotions we experience are signals.

Anxiety, for instance, is a signal that you believe that something bad is about to happen. When you have this thought, you will feel anxiety regardless of whether or not that prediction is accurate. When there is an objective threat, like you are about to be attacked by a bear, fear helps you escape from or confront danger as quickly as you can. The body kicks off an orchestrated response that includes increased heart rate, rapid breathing, and focused attention on the threat, so that you can manage the threat or get the heck out of there (the fight-or-flight response). Interestingly, the body doesn't differentiate a real threat from a false alarm. In other words, when you have the *perception* that there is impending doom, your body prepares you—it kicks off the fight-or-flight response—regardless of whether the threat is real. Think of a fire alarm. Pulling the fire alarm triggers a piercing sound irrespective of whether there is a fire. Your body does the same thing. It doesn't differentiate between a real threat and a perceived threat, which is also helpful. If you were on a hike and heard a sound in the bushes, you wouldn't want to take the time to ponder whether it was the wind or some predator; your body is wired to protect you and respond as if it's a real threat.

If you experience the emotion of anger, it's because you believe some injustice is occurring or someone has deliberately tried to offend or irritate you. For instance, you might believe that your partner's cutting words were an intentional slight or putdown. If you're frustrated, it's because you perceive that your expectations aren't being met or things aren't going as planned. Sadness often stems from thoughts about loss, disappointment, or unfulfilled needs.

You get the point—whenever you have an emotional experience, a thought is driving it. Emotions are important to understand because they let us know that there is something that needs to change—either how you are viewing the situation or what you can do about it.

Try to be aware of your emotions and use them as signals to pay attention to your thoughts. Whenever you notice your mood change toward your partner—for example, you're feeling more frustrated with them, angry, or, perhaps, hopeless about whether they will ever improve—that's your cue to pay attention. Ask yourself, "What is this emotion telling me? What messages am I telling myself based on this feeling?" Rather than reaching a conclusion right away and reacting to the emotion, see if you can look at it from another angle.

Understand and Shift Your Thinking

Our emotions are a signal that something needs to change—either we need to shift the way we view things or we need to take action to modify the circumstances. Here we'll focus on strategies for modifying your thoughts. The next chapter focuses on helping you change the situation.

Understanding and changing your thoughts will help you see things more clearly and respond in a way that will be more beneficial to you, your partner, and your relationship. Whenever you're feeling a negative emotion—like sadness, anxiety, frustration, or anger—use that as an opportunity to check out your thoughts. Ask yourself, "What was I thinking just before I started to feel this way?"

Often the thought will come in the form of a conclusion you may have reached about your partner's behavior or character. You might think your partner doesn't care about you, never listens or tries to understand, intentionally ignores you, is being selfish, is doing this to hurt you, isn't trying to get better, or is lazy and unmotivated. You might also have negative thoughts about the relationship itself: "We'll never get through this. This relationship is so one-sided. We have no emotional connection. We're just going through the motions."

Once you're aware of the thoughts contributing to your emotions, the next step is to treat them not as a foregone conclusion but as a possibility. In other words, it can be helpful to consider your thoughts hypotheses to be tested rather than facts. Ask yourself, "Am I viewing this situation as objectively as possible? What does the evidence tell me? Are there other ways of looking at this? Can I come up with a more neutral explanation than the one my brain defaults to? What would a friend say to me if they knew I had this thought? What would I say to a close friend if I knew they had the same thought?"

One way to have more balanced thoughts about your partner is to use a thought record. The same strategies discussed in Chapter 6 (about dealing with the thinking traps in depression) can be applied to thoughts you have about your partner.

TRY THIS: DEALING WITH NEGATIVE RELATIONSHIP THOUGHTS

On a piece of paper, your phone, or a tablet, briefly write down the situation (What happened when you became more negative about your partner?). What were the thoughts you experienced just before you started to feel this way? These are your automatic thoughts. What specific emotion were you feeling, and how intense was it from 0 (*not at all intense*) to 100 (*the most intense I have ever experienced*)? The table on pages 176–177 provides an example of Samantha's thought record.

Now that you have an idea of what you were feeling and thinking, review the evidence. What facts support the thought you had, and what facts don't support your thought? Try to stick to the facts rather than your interpretation of the facts. Once you have examined the evidence, the next step is to try to come up with a more balanced and helpful thought about your partner.

Finally, indicate how you are feeling now from 0 to 100. It's important to evaluate how you're feeling now to see whether changing the thought helped improve how you feel about your partner and the relationship. If it didn't, then it's important to investigate a little more. Might there be other thoughts that are driving how you are feeling that you haven't yet identified? Was the review of the evidence comprehensive enough, or did you miss some key facts? Was the alternative thought you came up with balanced? In other words, did the new thought incorporate all the evidence? It takes time and practice to learn how to catch, test, and change your thinking, but with a bit of time and effort, you will get there. If you want some additional step-by-step information on how to change your thinking, check out *Mind over Mood,* by Drs. Greenberger and Padesky.

Samantha (described at the beginning of this chapter) decided to complete a thought record about the thoughts she was having about Jack. Reviewing her thoughts and trying to balance them with evidence made her feel better and less negative toward Jack and the relationship (see the table on pages 176–177). It's important to note that the goal is to try to ground your thinking in facts as much as you can. This will help you develop alternative thoughts that are more balanced and proportionate to your experiences rather than being colored by tinted relationship glasses and negative partner schemas. This doesn't mean that the negative emotions will simply disappear. As you can see in the table, Samantha continued to feel some frustration, anger, sadness, disappointment, and hopelessness. What she experienced warranted these feelings; however, their intensity lowered when Samantha was able to see them in a more objective light. When we check out our thoughts and align them with facts and yet still experience negative emotions, we can add other strategies to our tool kit. Problem solving, communication, and acceptance strategies (reviewed in Chapters 13 and 14, respectively) may also help.

Samantha's Thought Record

Situation	Automatic thought	Mood/rating (0–100)	Evidence for the thought	Evidence against the thought	Balanced thought	Rerate mood (0–100)
Jack forgot to pick the kids up from school.	He's lazy.	Frustration 75	Jack spends a lot of time on the couch. He hasn't been helping much around the house.	Depression is legitimate and has zapped Jack's energy and motivation. He used to be active and helpful. Depression also impacts Jack's concentration.	Jack didn't mean to forget. It's not laziness—it's a symptom of his depression. He has a lot on his mind and is feeling overwhelmed.	40
Jack left his dirty laundry on the floor.	He doesn't care about me.	Sadness 85	Jack has often neglected the chores. He made a critical comment about me at dinner. I am doing more than my fair share of the housework and childcare.	Jack has been open with me about feeling numb and exhausted. He hugged me yesterday and apologized for not being himself.	Jack is struggling, and it's not a reflection of how much he cares. His actions are impacted by his depression, not a lack of love.	50
Jack forgot to pick up his prescription, and I ended up having to get it.	I'm the only one trying. He does nothing to help me or help himself.	Anger 90	I'm working, cleaning, cooking, parenting, and trying to support him emotionally. He is often forgetful.	Jack expressed feeling guilty and said he wants to get better. He went to therapy last week. He's helped around the house when his energy was better.	It feels lonely right now and hurts, but Jack is making some effort when he can. We're both hurting in different ways.	55

Jack and I sat and watched TV together. We didn't have much to say to each other.	We have no emotional connection.	Sadness 80	There are many times when we don't talk. We don't hug, kiss, or have sex as often as we used to. We don't say "I love you" as frequently.	We have had some good conversations when Jack is feeling more like himself. We are affectionate on occasion. Depression impacts Jack's energy and ability to engage. His medications have interfered with his sexual functioning.	Although we aren't as close as we used to be, I know that Jack still loves me. Depression is hard on both of us and makes it difficult to feel as connected as we used to. We do still have a connection; it's just strained for now.	45
Jack was on the couch scrolling on his phone.	We'll never get our relationship back. His depression won't change.	Disappoint-ment/ Hopelessness 80	Jack's been experiencing depression for quite some time. Our relationship has been strained.	Jack recently started seeing a psychologist for cognitive-behavioral therapy. He mentioned that it seems promising. Lately Jack has been making more effort to go for walks with me and trying to become more active. He has also tried to be more open with me. We have also experienced difficulties in the past and gotten through them.	Things are difficult right now, but the chances are good that Jack's depression will improve. Although depression has taken a toll on our relationship, we can get through this. There are glimmers of hope that our relationship can survive this turmoil.	20

Recall the Qualities That Initially Attracted You

Do you ever think back to when you met your partner? That initial glance from across the room or the first time you saw their profile on a dating app? Do you recall how the two of you met and what you talked about? Bring your mind back to the first month or two together. What was that like? Now, keeping your focus there, think about the qualities that first attracted you to your partner. What specifically excited you about them? What did you love about them? When you first told your friends about this great person you met, what did you say?

Thinking back to the qualities that first attracted you to your partner can be a powerful way to reconnect. It can also help shift your perspective and change the negative relationship glasses that you may have been wearing unwittingly.

In any long-term relationship, it's normal for the spark to fade over time. This is especially likely to happen when you're coping with the stress that accompanies partner depression. Recalling the positive qualities that first attracted you to your partner can help you see through the hurt, flaws, and disappointments. As you reflect on this, you might come to realize that these qualities are still there—they represent the core of who your partner is—but may have just gone underground for a bit or become stunted. Reflecting on these early memories might also rekindle affection for your partner.

Are you the sentimental type? Did you keep the cards and notes that your partner gave to you over the years? If so, you might want to dig them out. Perhaps they are stored in a memory box or a drawer. Take some time to read through them and relive the emotions you had when they were given to you. Although this might have an unintended effect of making you sad that things aren't what they used to be, it can also remind you who your partner is beyond the symptoms and the heartache you're currently experiencing. Try to focus on remembering those qualities that originally made you fall in love and use these positive memories to see your partner now.

It can be easy to think, "They were so kind and caring and funny, but now they are miserable, self-absorbed, and numb." If you are able, try to see this as a temporary state and have hope that these qualities will shine through again when the depression improves. It can also help to change the *but* to an *and. But*s tend to negate a statement; they cancel out what came before it. On the other hand, *and*s can incorporate two competing thoughts; they allow you to hold two seemingly disparate things in your mind at once such that both can be true. If you think "My partner says they love me, *but* doesn't show it the way I need," you could try rephrasing it as "My partner says they love me, *and* I wish they showed it more." "We enjoy time together, *but* we fight too much" can be changed to "We enjoy time together *and* we struggle." It may seem like semantics, but small shifts in what we tell ourselves and our partners can have a big impact on our willingness to connect and even forgive.

Notice Your Partner's Positive Behaviors

Remember the gorilla experiment, which demonstrated how easy it is to focus our attention on what we are expecting to see and ignore or negate information that doesn't fit? When we have negative partner schemas or tinted relationship glasses, it's so easy to see the faults in our partners and all the behaviors we dislike. At the same time, we can ignore the small (or even big) positives our partner is doing.

When we pay attention to the negative things and selectively ignore the positive, we can fall into another trap—making negative attributions. This happens when we see unwanted behavior as intentional or characteristic of our partner's personality and positive things as temporary or statelike. Earlier in this chapter we discussed how self-schemas can impact the attributions that individuals with depression make about themselves. When bad things happen, they attribute them to internal, stable, and global causes. When good things happen, they are seen as external, unstable, and specific. We can do the same thing when we evaluate our partner's behavior through negative relationship glasses. Let's say your partner does something you don't like. Our natural tendency in these circumstances is to think that the negative behavior is characteristic of them—part of their personality (they are lazy, unmotivated, they lack drive, and so on). Conversely, we're more inclined to view their positive behaviors as due to less stable factors. We see them as temporary and discount them. For example, rather than thinking that your partner folded the laundry or made you a cup of coffee because they are thoughtful, you might think they were simply in a good mood that day or were feeling guilty from the fight you had the night before.

You can improve how you feel about and respond to your partner by being aware of biases in attention and negative attributions used to explain their behavior. Try to train yourself to notice your partner's positive behaviors (and reinforce these). It may take some practice to learn to look for the positive things your partner does. Like Samantha and Jack, this takes little effort at the beginning of your relationship. In long-term relationships, however, it becomes more difficult to maintain. A natural tendency is to develop tinted glasses for our partners, especially when we have been hurt or gone through negative experiences. Start small and try to be deliberate in noticing the positive things your partner does. It's okay for it to be effortful.

Each day, ask yourself "What's one positive thing I can notice about my partner today?" (and write them down). If you can't think of anything, try to find even the tiniest example. They might have texted you during the day. You might recognize "They were thinking about me today." Maybe they made a joke or laughed at something funny you had said. Perhaps they asked how you slept last night, which shows they care and are checking in with you. These don't have to be big things but, the more you try to notice and pay attention to the positive things your partner is doing, the more you will tend to find. The more you find, the more your thinking will change about your partner.

You might even consider telling your partner what you have noticed. "You know, when you told me I looked nice when I was walking out the door this morning, that felt really nice" or "I really appreciated it when you helped me clean up the kitchen after supper. It made me feel cared for." Expressing your appreciation will help rekindle the relationship and allow you to remember that, amidst the pain and turmoil, there are positive qualities in your partner that you can bring out more by noticing and reinforcing. Over time, try increasing the positive things you notice.

Another strategy is to be aware of the attributions you're making about your partner. When they behave in a way you don't like, try to see it as a temporary blip and not characteristic of *who* they are. At this point, you might be saying to yourself, "But this isn't a *temporary* blip. This has been going on a long time." It's true that living with someone who is experiencing depression is exhausting and difficult. In this case, it might be helpful to at least see it as due to the depression rather than their personality. When your partner does positive things, try to see them as indicative of who they are and remind yourself that underneath that depression and misery is the person you first fell in love with. They are still there. They are just impaired in this moment, which makes it tremendously difficult to see. The more you can reinforce these positive behaviors the more likely they are to increase. Give it time. It will eventually get easier to retrain your brain to notice the good things and develop more neutral explanations for the bad.

As Drs. Nichols and Straus (2021) stated in their book *The Lost Art of Listening,* "You don't change relationships by changing other people. You change patterns of relationship by changing yourself in relation to them." When we work to change the way we think about our partners—to see them in a more positive (or at least non-negative) light—we feel better about our relationships. This, in turn, impacts how our partners respond to us.

Changing negative thinking about your partner isn't easy, especially if you've been wearing tinted relationship glasses for a long time. It takes a lot of awareness, effort, and practice. There will be some days when you will be better at it than others. And there will be days when you strike out. Just keep stepping up to the plate. Believe it or not, the baseball players who hit the most home runs also tend to be those who strike out the most.

13

Communication and Problem Solving

Ali's resentment had been building steadily. He loved Fatemeh deeply, but the weight of her sadness impacted their relationship and his own well-being. The constant negativity, blank stares, and broken plans had taken their toll. Ali was exhausted and about ready to throw in the proverbial towel. He was a problem solver and a fixer, but months of reading articles about depression, listening to podcasts, and consulting with friends and colleagues wasn't cutting it. Something had to change. He had been working diligently to complete thought records and keep his thinking in check (see Chapters 6 and 12), which helped him recognize that Fatemeh wasn't acting like this intentionally, and he learned not to take things personally. He also understood that her depression wouldn't last forever and tried not to lose hope. But feelings of anger and resentment remained. Their relationship needed other skills and resources to get them through this difficult time.

Jamie and Priya had been together for five years. Although many of those years were happy, Jamie had fallen into a deep depression over the last several months and the world seemed monochromatic and bland to him. Everything felt onerous. Although he hated to let Priya down, even a simple question like "How was your day?" made Jamie squirm. He felt overwhelmed. He didn't want to lie, but telling Priya the truth would, in his view, be too heavy and disheartening for her. Jamie recognized that Priya was doing her best to support him, but Priya seemed to be disengaging and that gnawed at him. She started going out more without asking if he wanted to join. He wouldn't have agreed to go, but not being asked felt like a blow and made him feel worse. Priya, on the other hand, tried to maintain a positive attitude and worked hard to reinterpret Jamie's behaviors in a more neutral light. She would tell herself that

Jamie was overwhelmed, not uninterested. That he was tired, not being cold and distant. But Priya felt like she was disappearing in the relationship. To her, being lonely in the relationship was worse than being alone. Something had to be done.

As discussed earlier (see Chapter 12), one way to enhance your relationship is for each of you to work at being evidence-based in how you think about the other. Your partner will likely have a tougher time with this because of the biases depression creates about self and others. Changing thinking about your partner or your relationship is powerful, but sometimes only gets you so far.

That doesn't mean you should give up on changing thinking. I would encourage you to keep at this. It's always a good idea to keep your thinking in check to make sure you're seeing things as objectively as possible. Decades of research have demonstrated that it can significantly improve your mood, help you manage stress and anxiety, and bolster your relationship. Over time, it will pay off. Examining your thoughts will help change your perspective about your partner and your relationship.

However, when you've aligned your thoughts with the facts and your mood still hasn't changed significantly, you may need to shift the focus toward what you can do about it.

Ask yourself, "Is there anything I can do to help improve the situation?" In this chapter, I suggest two things you can try to help change the situation and improve your relationship: (1) modify how you and your partner interact and (2) work alone or with your partner to resolve various problems and underlying issue(s).

Changing How You Communicate as a Couple

Many couples are effective at communicating early in the relationship, but communication breaks down over time. This is especially true when couples are dealing with mental health problems. Communication that was once positive and clear becomes negative and distorted. Intimacy seems like a distant memory and is replaced by pessimism and hopelessness.

Depression puts a strain on relationships; relationship distress, in turn, contributes to depression. Figuring out which is to blame is kind of like trying to ascertain whether the chicken or the egg came first—it's most likely a futile exercise. What is more productive is to maximize the odds that you and your partner communicate as effectively as possible, depression notwithstanding.

Keeping Tabs on Your Communication Style

A first step in making communication healthier is to take a mental inventory of where things are right now. How do you and your partner interact when you discuss relationship issues? Is one person typically more aggressive and the other more passive? Does one increase demands while the other withdraws? Do you bicker and escalate, or do you avoid and brush everything under the rug?

Sometimes couples resort to tactics like coercion because they haven't figured out a better way to get their relationship needs met. They may withhold affection, make threats that they will harm themselves or leave, or cry as a strategy for being heard or getting their way. This isn't necessarily even a conscious decision. Often, people aren't aware they are doing this. Although such strategies may work in the short term, they don't do anything to facilitate the relationship and, in fact, usually make problems worse. The partner on the receiving end of coercion often gives in just to make the demands stop. This inadvertently reinforces the unwanted behavior and can result in discontent, resentment, and anger.

Other unhealthy communication patterns can show up as well. For example, one partner may criticize the other, attacking their character or personality rather than focusing on the specific behaviors they would like to see changed. It's also easy to fall into the traps of showing contempt for a partner, hurling insults, and showing disrespect. Sometimes communication can break down because the response to a partner's concerns is met with defensiveness. They deny responsibility or shift the blame to their partner or someone else. Another common communication buster is stonewalling, where one person withdraws from the conversation and shuts down.

Try to be aware of how you're communicating with your partner and how your partner is communicating with you. Sometimes it can be helpful to remember that you're not enemies. Can you both agree to put a pause on the negativity and try a different approach?

Thinking about a recent interaction you had with your partner—an interaction that didn't go particularly well—can be a helpful exercise. Either alone or with your partner, think about where you each got stuck. Do a play-by-play and try to determine where things veered off course. Doing this can help you learn how you might revise your strategy so that the two of you can better connect and communicate.

If you have sat through intermission while watching a professional sport on television, you'll notice that broadcast teams do this all the time.

The commentary team provides insights and analysis about the game. Periodically, they will play part of a clip and freeze the play so they can help the viewer see what went wrong or what led to the collapse in defense, contributing to the opponent's goal, basket, or touchdown. Although memory can be fallible, you may be able to discover what you and your partner could have each done differently so that the conversation could have been more constructive.

Assuming that you and your partner are both invested in trying to resolve conflict and improve communication, the next step is to part ways with your default patterns of communication and adopt a different approach. This isn't easy, and it will take some practice, but over time you will feel understood, your partner will feel heard, and you will both be more likely to discuss issues in a way that allows you to see each other's perspective, meet in the middle, and resolve issues.

TRY THIS: SCHEDULING DISCUSSIONS USING THE SPEAKER AND LISTENER STRATEGY

Here's a strategy to help you and your loved one communicate better:

1. ***Set aside time when you are both ready.*** It's important to choose a time when you're both up to the challenge of discussing a problem or concern, such as when you aren't tired or hungry, and are in a state of relative calm (not in the heat of an argument).

2. ***Agree to take turns.*** One person will start as the Speaker and the other as the Listener. Figure out who will go first and come up with some ground rules, such as how long each person will have to speak (usually a minute or two) and what issue you will talk about.

3. ***Speaker rules.*** The Speaker expresses their concern using "I" statements (for example, "I feel frustrated that I am usually the one to initiate conversation," "I feel hurt that when I try to get close to you, you seem to pull away," or "I felt upset when you didn't call me or text me back"). The goal here is to express your feelings without getting riled up or into an argument. "You" statements usually result in the other person feeling blamed and attacked.

   It's also important to stick to one issue at a time. Try to focus on the behaviors or situation rather than making statements about your partner's character or personality. Be as concise and specific as possible.

4. ***Listener rules.*** The Listener's job is to, well, listen. But really listen. Try to understand and make your partner feel heard. Don't interrupt, respond, or start thinking about how you might respond. Instead, really zero in on what your partner is saying (see Chapter 2). Be aware of your body language while your partner is speaking and make sure you're being receptive to what they are saying. After the Speaker has finished, paraphrase what they have said to show your understanding. The Listener should summarize the Speaker's message without evaluating it or providing a response. And then check in to verify that the message was received accurately. For example, "What I heard you saying is ________. Did I get that right?"

5. ***Switch roles.*** Once you have each had an opportunity to be the Speaker or Listener, switch roles.

The goal in this exercise is to help each of you learn how to express your needs, desires, and concerns in a productive way that is less likely to lead to defensiveness or reactivity. Another objective is for you each to feel heard. When someone truly feels heard, they are more likely to respond in a way that will help address the concern and improve the relationship.

Ken and Carla planned for a time when they both felt calm to discuss what was concerning them about the relationship. Ken felt Carla was pushing him too much. He was deeply depressed and chronically fatigued and didn't have the energy or motivation to participate in activities, let alone plan and initiate them. Carla was frustrated. "It always lands on me to initiate the conversation or push for change. I feel like I'm always pressing forward, having to push for more." Carla was aware that Ken resented being pushed but was convinced he needed it. "If I stopped doing that," she said, "nothing would happen."

Ken was going to talk first (to be the Speaker). Carla's job was to be the Listener—to pay attention, demonstrate nonverbally that she was invested in the conversation, and let Ken express what he was going through. "I feel as though I am being pushed and nagged to do things and to get out more," Ken exclaimed. "I recognize you are trying to help, but I feel overwhelmed with the cards I have been dealt, and some days it's hard for me to do even simple things like getting out of bed and getting dressed." As Ken relayed his experience, Carla tried hard to listen and not interject. There were many times, especially at the beginning of the conversation, when she wanted to say "Yes, but" or provide a rebuttal. Although it was difficult, she found a way to really listen and not think of all the things she wanted to say in response. After Ken was finished, Carla summarized what she had heard and asked if she got it right.

It was then Carla's turn to play the role of the Speaker and for Ken to listen. After each person shared their perspective, Carla and Ken were in a better place to be able to move forward. They agreed they would have a signal for when Ken felt that Carla was pushing too hard. In this case, they used a hand gesture to indicate "stop." Carla would try to be more thoughtful in choosing when and how much she would "push" Ken. When she did urge Ken to act, she prefaced it in language of care and concern. At the same time, Ken agreed that he would do his best to initiate emotional intimacy and be more accessible and active when he was able. They heard each other, and, because they expressed their views in a calm, focused manner, they were more open to making changes that would benefit the other.

Assertiveness

Another strategy for getting your relationship needs met in a healthy and productive way involves assertiveness. Assertiveness means standing up for your rights in a way that is productive and confident without being passive or aggressive. When we are being passive, we are always putting others' needs before our own. At the extreme, this would be like being a doormat and letting others walk all over you. The belief when someone is passive is, "Your needs matter; mine don't." The flip side is being aggressive, where you only see your needs as the priority and don't consider others' needs. When someone is regularly aggressive, the belief is "It's a dog-eat-dog world. You gotta take care of number one." Assertiveness is squarely in the middle of these two extremes.

Being assertive means standing up for your own needs but in a way that respects others so that your responses are a win for both of you. The mentality of an assertive person is, "My needs matter and your needs matter."

The steps to being assertive are like the Speaker role described earlier: you want to be clear with yourself about what you specifically want. Once you are aware of your boundaries, needs, and feelings, express them using "I" statements. It's harder to get your back up when someone is speaking from how they are feeling and refraining from using accusatory language. As you are expressing what you need, be direct, confident, and specific. Try to remain calm. Listen to your partner's response and respect their point of view, but stand firm. Remember, it's okay to set boundaries and to say "no" without feeling guilty or having to overexplain why you feel the way you do. If your partner resists, try to restate your position calmly. If things escalate, take a pause and reintroduce the conversation again when things are less heated.

If you want to learn about strategies for being more assertive, Australia's Centre for Clinical Interventions has excellent resources (*www.cci.health.wa.gov.au/Resources/Looking-After-Yourself/Assertiveness*).

36 Questions

Good communication isn't always about learning to deal with conflict or issues that come up in a relationship. Sometimes it's about just getting to know your partner and spending time connecting. Dr. Arthur Aron, an internationally renowned relationship researcher, began testing out how couples can increase intimacy. He developed a list of 36 questions that cover a range of topics, from personal preferences and dislikes to ambitions and aspirations to personal values and vulnerabilities. The goal of these questions is to help members of a couple disclose to their partner information about themself that fosters closeness. Hundreds of studies have supported this idea. Another benefit is you may find these questions give structure to your conversations, which may be more difficult when your partner is depressed.

The concept went viral after a columnist featured this work in a *New York Times* story titled "To Fall in Love with Anyone, Do This." If you are interested in this research, you can catch a podcast on *Hidden Brain* called "Relationships 2.0: Keeping Love Alive," where host Shankar Vedantam interviews Dr. Aron (*www.hiddenbrain.org/podcast/relationships-2-0-keeping-love-alive*). To see the questions, visit *https://ggia.berkeley.edu/practice/36_questions_for_increasing_closeness.*

Problem Solving

When changing your thinking isn't getting you as far as you like, another helpful strategy is to problem-solve. Problem solving can be useful when there is something you can do to try to improve or remedy a situation.

Problem-solving strategies can help improve how you feel by figuring out how to best respond to a complex situation. This can help you feel less overwhelmed and offers a clearer path by which to deal with some of the difficult problems and emotions that arise when you are dealing with a partner's depression. You can use these techniques yourself or with your partner to solve problems together as a team.

The five main steps involved in problem solving are shown in the table below.

Kristen wrestled with the fact that she seemed to be doing all the work around the house. She recognized that this wasn't Mark's fault but needed to solve the problem since she remained frustrated and tired. Here's how she used IDEAS.

IDEAS for Problem Solving

Step	Definition
1. **I**dentify the Problem	Identify and define the problem as clearly as you can. Try to understand the problem from different perspectives.
2. **D**etermine the Options	Brainstorm as many solutions to the problem as you can.
3. **E**valuate the Options	Weigh the pros and cons of each option. See if you can come up with a solution that is most likely to improve the situation.
4. **A**ct	Once you have decided on a solution, try to implement it.
5. **S**ee If It Worked	After trying out your solution, take some time to evaluate how it went. Did this help make things better? Are you feeling less distressed by it? If so, great. If not, try to think of some other solutions.

Identify the Problem

Kristen wrote down, "I have to take care of everything because of Mark's depression. I am exhausted and overwhelmed." Then she gave it some more thought to provide a little more detail to really understand and nail down the specific problem. For instance, Kristen asked herself, "What specific tasks am I taking on? How much time does this take me? When I'm doing these tasks, how do I feel? Am I anxious because of everything else I need to do? Am I resentful?"

Determine the Options

Kristen came up with:

- Communicate more openly with Mark.
  - Without blaming Mark, express how I care and want to help but am feeling overwhelmed. See if Mark has some ideas about how I can help in ways that don't drain my tank.
- Set boundaries.
  - Have a conversation with Mark about what I am willing to do to help but also let him know that I can't manage everything on my own. Are there some things Mark could do to help share the responsibilities?
- Get some support.
  - I could look up a local support group, like the Depression and Bipolar Support Alliance. I could also think about individual therapy to help me through this. Couple therapy may be another option. Perhaps friends or family could help carry some of the responsibilities.
- Delegate responsibility.
  - I could come up with some ideas of what Mark could do to help, when possible—steps that won't overburden him, but may help him move him forward by taking small steps to be more active.
- Do things to recharge.
  - I could book time to visit with my friends or set up a schedule to ensure I have some downtime.

Evaluate the Options

Kristen noted that delegating responsibility might help Mark be more independent and give him a sense of accomplishment. It might also reduce the burden on Kristen. The main disadvantage may be that Mark declines or resists because depression has affected his energy and motivation. As you weigh the pros and cons of each solution, you're trying to find a solution that will meet your needs, will support your partner, and won't be too demanding. This helps you recognize that there is often more than one way to approach a problem and reduces the feeling of being stuck.

Act

Kristen decided to have a conversation with Mark about the need for some compromise: "I want to help support you as much as I can, but I have been feeling quite overwhelmed lately," she stated. "I wonder if we can come up with a plan where we start sharing more responsibility for some things. Maybe we can start with some smaller tasks and work our way up. What do you think?"

See If It Worked

Kristen took time to ask herself if things were moving in the right direction. "Mark has been able to take on some tasks. Has that helped reduce my load? Am I less overwhelmed or do I need to make some tweaks to this strategy? Are there other solutions to try out?" If the solution hasn't worked completely or there are new problems, adjust the plan. It can be an ongoing process, but by actively trying to problem-solve, you will feel more in control of the situation and develop ideas that will help you and your partner move forward.

Kristen also identified another problem: the lack of companionship in her relationship. Trying to **identify the problem** clearly, she came up with "I feel very alone in my relationship. I don't know how to connect with Mark. He feels distant, and I miss the closeness we used to share." On closer inspection, Kristen realized that she was both sad that she couldn't seem to reach Mark and frustrated that his depression was preventing them from interacting in meaningful ways. Kristen also had the thought "Mark doesn't care about my needs" (which might represent a thinking trap of catastrophizing or all-or-nothing thinking; see Chapter 6).

When Kristen worked to **evaluate the options,** she listed:

- Check out the evidence.
    - What makes me think that Mark doesn't care about my needs? What does the evidence say? Could it be that Mark's lack of emotional availability is more about his depression than about our relationship?
- Come up with other ways to connect.
    - Although the two of us aren't engaging emotionally like we used to, maybe there are small ways we can still connect. Maybe I could talk to Mark about how I feel or offer to sit together without pushing for there to be a conversation.

- Think about couple therapy.
- Consider support groups or individual therapy for me.

Weighing the pros and cons, Kristen decided to try one of the easier options first: checking out the evidence and coming up with other small ways to connect with Mark. Couple therapy was an option that Kristen put in her back pocket for now. Although it could help improve communication and intimacy, a downside was that Mark may not be open to the idea at this point.

Kristen followed the next step—**act**—by examining some of the thoughts she was having, looking at whether she was falling into some thinking traps, and coming up with more helpful, alternative thoughts. She also decided to have a conversation with Mark (using the Speaker-Listener technique). During this conversation, Kristen expressed her desire for closeness and inquired whether she and Mark could work together to reconnect in small but tangible ways. Kristen suggested finding small, low-pressure ways to connect, like texting each other more throughout the day, doing some fun activities together, and spending more time together (even if it was in silence).

Then Kristen evaluated the outcome to **see if it worked.** After giving it some time, she considered whether these steps had helped them feel closer or if there was still a palpable distance between Kristen and Mark that was nagging at her. She knew that, if the issue hadn't been resolved satisfactorily, she could try other strategies to connect with Mark. Eventually Kristen recommended that they see someone for couple therapy: "I know you're going through a tough time, and I want to be here for you. But I also need to feel more connected with you. I wonder if therapy might help us with this?"

These steps can help break down some of the complex emotional challenges you are experiencing into manageable steps. They might give you more of a sense of control over difficult circumstances and allow you to get your needs met in a way that doesn't jeopardize your relationship.

As mentioned earlier, you can use problem-solving strategies as a couple as well, working together as a team. For instance, you might want to apply the IDEAS steps to discuss financial issues, figure out how to best manage the kids, address communication breakdowns, handle household responsibilities during and after the depression, deal with emotional connectedness and intimacy, or make major life decisions.

The key in problem solving is that you (and your partner) adopt an attitude that the stress and problems you face are solvable—to view them as a challenge to be conquered rather than as a threat to be avoided. Try to approach this as a team, focusing outwardly on resolving the issues you are confronting as a couple. You aren't enemies. You're a team. You can handle this together.

Communication and problem solving take time, effort, and patience. If you and your partner have given it a try and it didn't quite go as expected, don't give up. Take a break and, if you are both willing, revisit it again later. With practice, you can get better at it and your relationship can improve as a result. If you find that this is an impossible task for you right now, that's okay too. Let it go for now. There may be a time when you will want to come back to it or perhaps you need some more intensive help learning these strategies through couple therapy.

So far, we have focused on how to improve your relationship by targeting negative thinking, communicating differently, and solving relational problems independently or as a couple. There may also be times when what you are dealing with doesn't seem changeable. In these circumstances, we need to shift our attention to acceptance, which is discussed next.

14

Acceptance Strategies

Jonathan met Peter at a friend's barbecue. Although he was very attractive, what really stood out to Jonathan was Peter's quiet confidence. He listened more than he spoke and seemed content to observe others from outside the group. When Peter did contribute to the conversation, it was thoughtful and insightful. Peter wasn't trying to impress anyone, and Jonathan appreciated that.

Throughout their relationship, Jonathan was emotionally demonstrative, whereas Peter was measured and consistent. He was always the steady one—calm, cool, and collected. This didn't irritate Jonathan at first, but after a while he started to view Peter as overly reserved and closed off. Peter was a private person and kept his cards close to his chest. That bothered Jonathan, especially after Peter became depressed and started to withdraw even more. When Jonathan asked him how he was doing, Peter just shrugged or said, "I'm fine." He knew Peter wasn't "fine," and it bothered Jonathan that he wouldn't tell him what was really going on.

One evening, after pouring a couple of glasses of wine on the back deck, Jonathan mustered the courage to raise his concerns. "I feel like you don't let me in," he said. "I never know *what's going on inside your head.*" Peter tried to defend himself. "I have never been one to wear my heart on my sleeve, Jonathan. You know that. I'm not sure what you want me to say." Jonathan had always hoped for a relationship where they shared emotions honestly and openly. He wanted emotional curiosity and expression. But Peter was naturally reserved and self-contained, even before the depression. Jonathan assumed that Peter would share more of his true feelings, once they built enough trust in the relationship, but that wasn't Peter's personality. It never was. The more Jonathan pushed for change, the more Peter resisted and the more disillusioned Jonathan felt in the relationship.

When we're upset with certain qualities, characteristics, or behaviors of our partners, we often focus a great deal of attention and effort on trying to change them. We may raise these concerns gently in conversation—or not so gently during arguments—hoping they will change. We pour our energy into "helping" them change, only to find that they aren't able or willing. Nothing seems to work. We feel stuck, and negative feelings intensify.

Rather than refining our strategies, we continue to push and prod, hoping that a particular characteristic or behavior will change. We refuse to let go. Because, if we do, we fear resigning ourselves to a relationship that won't be satisfying or ever measure up to our expectations and standards. Bitterness and resentment creep in, and we become more entrenched in our stance. Meanwhile, our partners aren't changing, and the relationship gets polarized.

Aligning *with* Your Partner

If you have gotten caught up in a struggle of trying to change your partner and seem to be hitting a wall, you might want to try focusing on emotional acceptance—different strategies that will help increase mutual understanding and empathy to align *with* your partner rather than working *against* them.

Hearing Your Partner's Heart, Not Just Their Voice

When your partner has been depressed for a long time, there is often a lot of emotional pain—scars from things that were said, hurts from feeling let down, resentments about their lack of progress or unwillingness to try the next treatment. When we express our hurt, we can often use an accusatory tone and blame our partners, pointing out their flaws or how they have frustrated or angered us. Not surprisingly, this typically leads to defensiveness and counterattacks.

Hearing the heart can be a powerful relationship builder that allows each of you to express what you are feeling without accusation. This involves a shift from what your partner did or didn't do to expressing the hurt you are experiencing. It means *feeling with* each other rather than fixing, judging, or defending. Doing so makes you more likely to move toward greater connection, compassion, and understanding.

You and your partner might be very aware of emotions you both express. You might be less aware of the hidden feelings and thoughts that underlie the problem. Thoughts of guilt, for example, that you somehow contributed to your partner's problem or feelings of sadness that you don't feel connected the way you used to. These thoughts and emotions are often not expressed because we are so focused on the immediate infraction, and more dominant emotions take over.

Whenever there is a hard emotion, like anger or resentment, there is usually an underlying soft emotion that coincides with it—an emotion that speaks to feelings of vulnerability and hurt. Being aware of the soft emotions that underlie the hard emotions you express can facilitate communication and understanding within the relationship.

If you express anger that your partner is always on their phone, underneath there might be a softer, more vulnerable emotion like sadness that you feel invisible or that it doesn't seem as though you are a priority in their life. When you express anger that you always have to do everything, you might also be experiencing a softer emotion, like "I want to feel like we're a team. I am exhausted and overwhelmed."

We are all more likely to be responsive to soft than hard emotions. It's difficult to become defensive and cranky when soft emotions and vulnerability are communicated. Revealing soft emotions opens your partner to joining forces with you to find other ways to tend to your needs.

The key to hearing the heart is to align with your partner and for both of you to express vulnerability. Instead of feeling like enemies, you start to be able to see each other in a light that exudes empathy, compassion, and acceptance. You could use the same approach as the Speaker-Listener strategy (see Chapter 13), only this time you are explicitly sharing some of the soft emotions (loneliness, sadness, fear, guilt, shame) that you are experiencing that may get buried because they are covered up by hard emotions (anger, frustration, blame).

Sharing from the heart can create a sense of mutual empathy where you recognize you are both hurting and may be open to finding ways to speak more gently and act with more compassion for each other. When you approach each other with empathy, you'll be less defensive and more likely to side with your partner's view (and they with yours), resulting in reciprocal understanding and care. This is an important way to build emotional acceptance.

Making the Problem (Not Your Partner) the Enemy

Whenever there is conflict and friction in a relationship, it's easy to point fingers at each other and get stuck in blame mode: "You never listen. You're always defensive. You never think about anyone but yourself. You don't even try." The conversation can easily become *me* versus *you*.

Instead of seeing an issue as caused by your partner, it can help to see the problem as something you can team up against and tackle together. In other words, you might be able to view the problem as an "it." In this way, the *problem* (not the couple) becomes the enemy and dealing with it becomes a shared challenge. Sometimes giving the "enemy" a name can help. For example, rather than saying, "You're so critical," you could recognize that "criticism shows up in our conversations a lot. Can we try to figure out a way to reduce it?" Instead of stating, "You only care about your work," you could team up against the real issue by recognizing that "It seems as though time has been hard to manage for both of us. We seem to be stuck in a pattern where work is taking over." The problem then becomes a challenge that both of you can solve together, which enhances emotional acceptance. For instance, you could organize your schedules at the beginning of the week to ensure that you schedule time together.

Another way to do this is to view your differences as stemming from your unique backgrounds (such as how you each grew up, cultural or gender differences). Peter (described earlier) grew up in a home where it wasn't okay to express emotions openly. His parents both kept a stiff upper lip and learned to grin and bear problems rather than talking about them. Jonathan, on the other hand, grew up in an emotionally expressive family. These respective styles put a strain on their relationship and worsened with Peter's depression. Jonathan and Peter eventually stopped blaming each other and started to view their communication styles as differences rather than deficiencies. They started to empathize and work with each other's communication style. The differences in communication became the "it" that they worked through together, an adversary they could both face.

TRY THIS: MAKING THE PROBLEM AN "IT"

Take time as a couple to consider whether you and your partner are treating each other as the problem. Can you shift your perspective to view the real issue as a challenge (instead of a threat) you can both deal with? Try to name the problem or issue, without getting into blaming or criticizing. Then view it objectively as a puzzle to be solved (see Chapter 1) and talk about how the problem is affecting you and impacting your interactions. Speaking from the heart will trigger less conflict or defensiveness. What is "it" doing to us? And, importantly, what would it take for us to tackle this problem together rather than blaming each other?

Emotional acceptance is really at the heart of what we want in a relationship—to be our true selves, vulnerable with our partners, knowing they accept us as we are (and that they are truly accepted for who they are, warts and all). When we can tap into this and make this a focus, our relationship burden can lift significantly.

Acceptance

Insisting on change makes sense at times. If communication is lacking, or there is regular conflict, figuring out strategies to improve interactions or resolve disagreements can be beneficial. Similarly, if your partner's depression is negatively affecting the relationship, there are strategies you can try to minimize the impact. But some things can't change easily.

Whenever we experience a painful event, like working through the anguish of a partner's depression, we tend to want to understand, fix, or get rid of it. Although these strategies may help, they often backfire.

Consider the Chinese finger cuffs. If you have never seen them, Chinese finger cuffs (or finger traps) are hollow cylinders made of thin strips of bamboo or some other flexible material. They are about five or six inches in length and one inch in diameter, just wide enough to insert a finger into each end. When you try to pull your fingers out, the woven structure contracts and grabs your fingers more firmly. The more you pull, the tighter it gets. The way out of Chinese finger cuffs is to gently push your fingers in toward each other. When you do this, the tension loosens, and you can slip your fingers out.

Much like the Chinese finger cuffs, the more we try to control, wrestle with, or overanalyze our problems the harder it can be to find a resolution. Sometimes the best way out is to move toward the discomfort (like the fingers) and accept what we are experiencing. Trying to push away distress or pain often amplifies it and pulls you further into a negative loop where it takes over and becomes your central focus.

Understanding the pain you're experiencing can certainly be helpful at times, and this is where changing your thinking (see Chapter 12) and problem solving (see Chapter 13) come in. By examining our thoughts, we put ourselves in a good position to know whether our thinking may be biased and unhelpful or is accurate and proportional to the situation. When our thoughts are accurate and distress remains, problem solving is often valuable for figuring out what to do. However, sometimes the distress we are experiencing doesn't improve by shifting our thoughts or finding a "solution." Sometimes a situation isn't fixable or changeable. In these situations, we often try to push the negative feelings aside and ignore or avoid them. That doesn't help either.

An old psychological experiment demonstrates how pushing a thought away only makes it more powerful. Participants were told to think of anything they wanted but to not think of a white bear. Those individuals who were asked *not* to think of a white bear ended up thinking about it a lot, even more than those who were instructed to think of a white bear. The reason for this finding is that trying to suppress our thoughts doesn't work. In fact, it makes the thought come back stronger and more frequently. When we experience pain, distress, and negative emotions and we try to push them away, they rebound and start to eat away at us. Meanwhile, living life is pushed aside.

Acceptance doesn't mean resignation, hopelessness, or defeat. Acceptance is about acknowledging that, although some things—like your partner's depression—are beyond your control, you can maintain the power to choose how to respond.

The well-known Serenity Prayer, used in Alcoholics Anonymous, is a reminder of the importance of discerning when change strategies might be helpful and when it's better to focus on acceptance:

God, grant me the serenity

to accept the things I cannot change,

courage to change the things I can,

and wisdom to know the difference.

You will likely face times when you have done all you can to manage your thoughts and emotions, and you're still feeling distressed. When there is nothing tangible you can do to try to change your thoughts or the situation, you might consider acceptance.

To illustrate, someone grappling with physical pain may try various strategies to alleviate their discomfort. Pain medications, used judiciously, may reduce pain. Physical therapy can deal with some of the causes of pain and improve the experience. Psychological treatments, such as cognitive-behavioral therapy, help manage pain. But sometimes an individual might be in chronic pain and, regardless of the interventions, still experience considerable discomfort. In these situations, accepting the pain might be a way out. Acceptance won't eliminate the pain, but it will help someone minimize catastrophizing about the pain experience and reduce the chance of making things worse. Acceptance can help someone both be in pain *and* continue to live despite the pain. The same is true for psychological pain and pain in relationships.

Instead of fighting against your feelings or pushing for change, you might decide to accept the pain and frustration. It may seem contradictory, but (like the Chinese finger traps) doing so can help reduce anxiety and emotional strain, find peace within difficult circumstances, and provide clarity in how to move forward.

This doesn't mean being okay with things that need to change. We do need to set limits and establish boundaries in a relationship. But it's being open to the fact that this is how things are right now. Accepting the truth of what is. When you can learn to accept what you are going through, you are more open to moving in the direction of living according to your values without being bogged down with repetitive thinking about changing the other person in your life.

Dr. Steve Hayes developed an approach to psychotherapy called Acceptance and Commitment Therapy. In one of his books, Hayes uses the metaphor of an unwelcome guest. Let's say you sent out an invitation to your local community to join you at your home for a party. Many people show up, including that one person in the community you despise. They are rude, obnoxious, and untrustworthy. You don't want them at your home, but what do you do? It was an open invitation to everyone in the community. You now have a choice. You can dwell on the fact that this person is at your party and lament about how awful it is. You can keep focused on this individual and follow them into every room of your house, making sure that they don't double-dip, swear, offend others, act inappropriately, or steal your stuff. In this case, you won't enjoy a single minute of the party. Your entire focus would be on the unwelcome guest.

Alternatively, you can accept that they are there. You don't have to like it, but by accepting it you can get on with the party. Your attention is no longer focused on *their* behavior; it's focused on enjoying the party.

Acceptance doesn't mean you need to like it. It's recognizing that this just is the way things are right now. Rather than judging it, trying to push it away, or attempting to fix it, you let it be. You accept that these are the cards you were dealt and deliberately decide to live *with* the problem: "Even though I don't like it, I am going to accept, for now, that this is my experience and move forward with living life, even while distress is here." Your partner's depression is real. Sometimes it's not possible to "fix" it. But this doesn't mean you need to give up on the relationship or resign yourself to a life of emotional distance.

You might be surprised. The act of letting go might go a long way in helping you manage your emotions.

What Kinds of Things Should I Learn to Accept?

Sometimes it's important to step back and recognize what is worth accepting about our partners rather than trying to change. Here are a few examples of things that are difficult, if not impossible, to change:

- ***Core personality.*** Whether your partner is more introverted or extroverted will not change. Similarly, your partner's sense of humor, their typical enthusiasm and energy for social gatherings, their need for space, or their sensitivity will not likely change dramatically. These characteristics represent who they are as individuals.
- ***Ability to process emotions or intellectual curiosity.*** Not everyone thrives on deep emotional connection, and your partner's ability to reveal their emotions is also not likely to change significantly over time. Some people need time to process what they are experiencing whereas others want to talk it out instantly. Although it can be productive to work on your communication styles, there are likely aspects that you won't be able to change. This may not match your style, and that's okay. Similarly, not everyone needs to feel stimulated intellectually, whereas others crave this. These differences, which are not likely to change, might be better to accept.
- ***Need for independence/togetherness.*** Some people need time on their own to reenergize and collect their thoughts. Others crave closeness and want to be together all the time. These tendencies often don't change much.
- ***Sex drive.*** You and your partner might experience differences in how frequently you crave sexual intimacy. It is common for there to be differences in sex drive. They may never align perfectly with your expectations and desires. Drive isn't something you can control. Although it's important to compromise, a dose of acceptance might help you navigate these differences.
- ***Annoying habits.*** There may also be things your partner does that you find annoying but aren't dealbreakers. Although you might be able to come up with some ways to minimize these irritations, it's important to pick your battles. Sometimes, the best course of action might be to just tolerate and accept these habits rather than constantly trying to change them.

When you have negative thoughts about your partner, ask yourself, *Is this changeable, and is it worth trying to change? If so, have I done everything I can to improve the situation?* If it is not changeable, it isn't worth trying to change, or you have tried everything and it's fallen flat, you may want to give acceptance a try. Whenever something is outside of your personal control, accepting it may be the better strategy. By allowing it to be there, without trying to change or get rid of it, the problem won't consume your attention. Once you have learned to accept your partner's depression, personality, or characteristics you don't care for, you will be freer to live a life that is consistent with your goals and values without being bogged down with the pain and suffering.

Live According to Your Values (as an Individual and a Couple)

Once you have tried acceptance strategies, you might also want to step back and view your partner and relationship from a wider perspective.

Viewing your partner and your partner's behaviors from a distance can make them feel less damaging and less urgent to resolve. Think of the difference between standing outdoors in the center of a storm and watching a weather report about it on television. Same storm, but with much less impact on you. It's hard to see beyond your immediate relationship struggles. But as you try to see it from a different perspective—to obtain greater emotional distance—you become more able to reflect on your issues objectively and connect the dots better. Stepping back even further allows you to see an even bigger picture. Although it's not easy to gain this distance and objectivity, it can help you understand your struggles and make sense of the larger story of you and your partner.

One way to step back and gain a wider perspective is to think about your values as an individual, as a partner, and as a couple. Values are what you consider most important in your lives. They refer to who you want to be and the ideals you aspire to. Values are not goals that we achieve; they are ways in which we live. They can help us view our relationships from the bigger picture (the satellite images) and can guide our decisions and actions. When we act in a way that is aligned with our values, we experience a sense of purpose and motivation. When we are misaligned with our values, we can feel uncomfortable and unsatisfied.

TRY THIS: IDENTIFYING YOUR RELATIONSHIP VALUES

Take a moment to think about what values you want to live by in your relationship. To be kind, compassionate, and understanding? Is loyalty, tolerance, or forgiveness core to your value system? Is dependability, honesty, and respect key? Who do you want to be as a partner? What values are important to your relationship?

Imagine you're having your 50th wedding anniversary. You've decided to rent a banquet hall and invite your friends and family. The place is decorated exquisitely. There are pictures of the two of you posted on the walls. Balloons and streamers line the ceiling. Tables are covered in fine linen, candles, and the same types of flowers you had in the wedding bouquet. Now imagine that each person at the celebration is going to make a toast and talk about what you are like as a couple and as individuals in the relationship.

What characteristics and values would you want people to mention? Write some of these qualities down. This is what is important for you to live by even while you are dealing with difficulties of partner depression.

Once you have identified your values (which you can do independently or with your partner), plan for how you are going to start putting this into action. Try to commit to exercising these qualities. How will you respond to your partner and act in a way that aligns with your core values? This doesn't have to involve massive changes. It's about starting small and building from there: "Today, I am going to try ________ so that I can get a little closer to where I want to be in my relationship."

Couples can be so focused on their current problems or what needs to change that they forget to think about their relationship as a whole and what they really want their relationship to be about.

By understanding your values, you will be able to take deliberate action toward supporting them. When we're hurt, angry, or defensive, it's easy to get caught up in the moment. But adopting a wider lens and seeing what really matters to us in the long run can create a healthy space between our emotions and how we end up responding to them. You will be more likely to respond than react. If you value respect, you might pause before snapping back when your partner seems irritable. If curiosity is an important value, you might ask yourself, "What's really going on with them?" instead of making assumptions.

Within a year of moving in together, Maria noticed that Leszek was not well. He seemed to stare blankly into space and rarely said a word. She learned how to connect first (see Chapter 2) and not fix things. Maria kept thinking, "If I just say the right thing . . . love him better . . . help him see . . . then maybe things will turn around." She tried everything possible and nothing seemed to work. She longed for the relationship she once had.

Maria was exhausted not only from the extra duties she took on while Leszek was going through depression, but also from trying to change what she couldn't. Maria started to wonder if this stagnation in her relationship was the way it was always going to be.

One afternoon Maria met a friend for lunch and relayed her distress. Her friend replied, "What if the goal isn't to get back to how your relationship was, but to learn how to love each other even with the pain and heartache—with what's going on for you both right now?" That resonated with Maria. Over the next couple months, she focused on letting go of control. She worked to love Leszek with his depression, not fighting incessantly against it. Doing this helped Maria feel less frantic and more grounded. She was no longer bitter or resentful, just present with what she was facing one day at a time. Maria never gave up. It wasn't surrender or resignation; instead, she worked on allowing what was. It meant that she could grieve the relationship she imagined having, accepting that this is the way things are at right now, and maintaining hope that the relationship could still grow. Hope, for Maria, came not from pushing change but from accepting and working with the relationship she had with Leszek in the present moment. This allowed her to feel more compassion both for Leszek and for herself.

At times, our problems can be magnified because we focus so much on trying to push them away, manage the pain, or change the situation. Our minds are so focused on changing our circumstances that we sometimes forget that some things aren't changeable (or worth pushing for change), at least in the moment. Constantly trying to change the unchangeable makes us more miserable because our thoughts are always oriented toward the possibility rather than the present. There are things that you can't change about your partner. In these instances, acceptance is key.

Adding acceptance to your repertoire will likely help you feel better. It will also likely help improve your interactions with your partner. We so easily fall into the trap of trying to change the other person's behavior when a more helpful strategy might be to just align with our partners, adopt a wider perspective, accept what we cannot change, and live according to our core values.

PART FOUR

The Final Word

15

When Your Partner Improves (or Doesn't Improve)

Congratulations for making it this far. By reading this book, you have gained new strategies to help your partner, support yourself, and improve your relationship. You have stuck it out and learned about the nature of depression, how to connect first, and support your partner in the ways that resonate best with them. You have gained information about effective evidence-based treatments and strategies for encouraging your partner to seek help. You read about how to support your partner to engage in antidepressant behavior and manage negative thinking. And you have thought about some of the more difficult aspects of handling depression and managing this turmoil.

The journey likely hasn't been easy. And it may continue to be a struggle. It's emotionally and physically exhausting and takes a lot of patience, compassion, and hard work.

You also learned how to keep yourself psychologically healthy throughout the chaos and how to work on your relationship when your partner is depressed.

I hope you've found many of the strategies offered in this book helpful, but please keep trying the ones that may not have been as immediately useful. Don't give up. Continue to have hope. The techniques described in this book are based on the best evidence available. They may not all work for everyone, but they represent important strategies for managing this difficult part of your life.

If you ever do find yourself beginning to lose hope, reach out to others for support and be gentle with yourself. Even take a break from using the techniques and go back to implementing them when you have rested, had some space, and taken a few deep breaths.

It's important to remember that there is no quick fix for depression. It would be nice if there was, but getting over depression and staying depression-free typically takes a lot of work. Even specialized psychological treatments, like CBT, typically take 12 to 16 sessions (and sometimes longer, depending on the severity and other complicating factors). So, be patient. Your partner will likely improve over time.

Preventing Relapse/Recurrence

If your partner has improved and their depression has subsided, wonderful. I am sure you're relieved. Hopefully you have now gotten to a point where you are able to focus more on yourself and your relationship and feel more connected with your partner. If this represents your situation, breathe a sigh of relief and celebrate the victory. Savor the moment.

However, now wouldn't be the time for either of you to let your guard down. Depression tends to reemerge. As discussed earlier in the book, the odds of experiencing future episodes of depression increase with each episode. Given this, it would be prudent to think about some strategies for preventing relapse or recurrence.

There is no one cure-all for preventing relapse and staying well. The best bet is to continue using a variety of strategies that will help your partner flourish and reduce the risk that depression will come back. It's almost like tending to a garden. By keeping up with the weeds before they spread and maintaining a watchful eye for critters that might harm the plants, you can manage a garden well. Similarly, your partner can increase their odds of staying depression-free by being aware of risk factors and engaging in things like psychological treatment, keeping thinking in check, behavioral activation, and healthy lifestyle habits. These elements are like the sunlight, water, and soil a garden needs to thrive.

Many of the best ways to prevent depression from worsening or returning are outlined in this book. As such, one good strategy is to revisit different chapters and work together to keep on top of, or brush up on, these skills.

Here are some additional tips for preventing relapse:

1. ***Evidence-based psychological treatment.*** Cognitive-behavioral therapy (CBT), behavioral activation, and interpersonal psychotherapy are well-researched treatments that not only effectively treat depression but

significantly reduce the risk of relapse. If your partner hasn't tried one of these treatments, it might be worth considering.

2. ***Booster sessions.*** Therapists often offer booster sessions for clients, after they have improved, to reduce the risk of relapse. They can be scheduled flexibly. For example, your partner could decide to see their psychologist or other regulated mental health professional once a month at first. These sessions can then be spread apart to every three months or every six months, for instance. I sometimes see clients once a year for mental health "checkups." These sessions can be helpful to keep up the skills learned and get a psychological tune-up. Although many people find booster sessions helpful, research isn't entirely clear that they are necessary to stay well.

3. ***Keep up with behavioral activation.*** To the extent your partner can keep up with behavioral activation (see Chapter 5), they will improve their odds of staying depression-free. Doing things that provide a sense of pleasure and accomplishment provides joy and purpose, which are antidepressant. The more these activities can involve connecting with others, the better. A sense of connectedness and mattering is super important to mental health and well-being.

4. ***Continue to keep thinking in check.*** Depression and negative thinking go hand in hand. An effective way to keep depression at bay is to ensure that your partner's thoughts are grounded in evidence (see Chapter 6).

5. ***Medication.*** If your partner has been on antidepressant medications, it is wise to stay on them for a period (usually 6–12 months). Research has demonstrated that this reduces the risk of relapse. They should consult with their family physician or psychiatrist to determine the best approach for continuance or maintenance medication.

6. ***Consider mindfulness-based cognitive therapy.*** Mindfulness-based cognitive therapy (MBCT) is an evidence-based approach shown to reduce the risk of relapse in individuals who have experienced three or more past episodes of depression. This approach helps keep thinking present-focused (rather than on the past or the future) by learning mindfulness practices (like breathing meditation) and strategies to disengage from negative thought patterns.

7. ***Distinguish sad mood from relapse.*** Your partner can easily get pulled into depression when they worry and ruminate about being sad. It's important to remember that negative emotions are a signal that we need to do

something (see Chapter 12)—they help us solve problems. Many people who have experienced depression worry that it will return and tend to catastrophize as soon as they experience any sadness. Understanding the difference can be helpful. You and your partner don't want to ignore symptoms of depression, but having some off days is a normal part of life.

8. ***Create a plan to stay well.*** Just as people might come up with a plan for maintaining physical conditioning, deriving a strategy for staying in mental shape can be beneficial. Part of this involves learning from experience. Think about what things might have originally triggered your partner's depression. Can they prepare for handling things differently should this stress come up again? Anticipate problems and setbacks and come up with a game plan. It might also help for your partner to keep a journal while well so that if a relapse does occur in the future, their own words can give them hope that it does get better.

9. ***Be on the lookout.*** What signs could you notice that might suggest your partner is slipping into depression again? For some, it's their sleep habits; for others, you might notice negative thinking or social withdrawal. Be on the lookout for these things (but try not to be hypervigilant. You are looking for a pattern, not isolated incidents—see point 7).

10. ***Lifestyle changes.*** Think about what lifestyle changes helped your partner feel better. We know that good nutrition, sleep, and exercise are important, for example. It's also helpful to minimize alcohol or other substance use. Stress is also a trigger for relapse. Your partner may want to learn strategies like relaxation or problem solving so that they don't feel so overwhelmed when confronted with stress.

Couple Interventions

Whether it's best for your partner to see a professional for depression in individual therapy or engage in couple therapy is a difficult decision. It depends, in part, on whether the relationship distress preexisted the depression. If your relationship was humming along until depression put a major strain on it, then treating the depression may also improve your relationship. In cases where relationship problems existed before, treating the depression will help your partner feel better but is not likely to fully address the issues in your relationship. In other words, relationship problems will likely continue even when your partner's depression lifts.

If you and your partner are experiencing relationship difficulties, you may want to see someone for couple therapy who also specializes in treating depression. Research suggests that couple-based interventions that focus on depression are effective in reducing both relationship distress and depression.

Numerous techniques for boosting your relationship were provided in this book. However, if you continue to struggle to reconnect, renegotiate roles, or regain intimacy, you might want to consider couple therapy. You can think of it almost like the difference between do-it-yourself projects and getting professional help. Taking care of things on your own may make sense in certain circumstances. However, there are also times when bringing in the skilled professional makes the most sense (see Chapter 4). Couple therapy can help resolve conflict, deepen connection, improve communication, and navigate various challenges.

Although there are many good options to choose from, three evidence-based approaches to couple therapy are (1) integrative behavioral couple therapy, which helps couples learn strategies to increase emotional acceptance (see Chapter 14) and change problematic behaviors in the relationship that are causing distress; (2) cognitive-behavioral couple therapy, in which couples learn to analyze and change the thoughts and beliefs that contribute to problems in their relationship; and (3) emotion-focused therapy, which focuses on strengthening emotional connection and identifying negative interaction patterns that are rooted in unmet emotional needs. These approaches have excellent research support behind them and are effective for couples in which one partner experiences depression.

Forgiveness

After going through so many difficulties associated with your partner's depression, you may experience residual resentment or anger for some of the negative experiences and emotions you've endured. At the same time, your partner may have unresolved feelings about some of the misunderstandings, impatience, or frustration that were expressed by you. Forgiveness is a healthy way to ease the pain and suffering caused by these negative experiences.

Putting the anger, sadness, hurt, and resentment aside and responding with empathy, mercy, and compassion will enable you to move forward in your relationship. Forgiveness means working through the pain and accepting what happened—the emotional distance, withdrawal, irritability, or periods of neglect you experienced. By doing so, you will be able to understand how the painful circumstances of your partner's depression unfolded and see it from their perspective.

When my kids were young, my daughter did something that upset my son. When she asked for forgiveness, my son, who was only about five years old at the time, said, "It's not okay, but I forgive you." What a wise statement from such a young child. Forgiveness is about having the resolve to let it go, see it as water "under the bridge," and move on. It involves a deliberate choice to repair trust and reestablish intimacy. Forgiveness doesn't make the infraction fair or excusable, and it's not about brushing it aside and pretending the hurt didn't happen. *It's not okay, but I forgive you.*

These may be difficult conversations to have and even tougher emotions to get over. You might have felt unappreciated or exhausted from carrying more than your fair share of the responsibilities. You may continue to feel mad about what depression did to your relationship and your life. These feelings are valid. Forgiveness, however, will help you move on without harboring resentment. It will allow you to grieve what you lost during this period and, at the same time, empower you both to regain intimacy and provide growth opportunities for your relationship.

There may be instances when you want to seek forgiveness from your partner as well. They may be hurting from all that unfolded during their depression. There may have been critical comments (intended or not), ridicule, or thoughtless acts. Seeking forgiveness can also lift a burden for you and help rekindle your relationship.

Finally, you may also need to get to a point where you forgive yourself. Let go of the guilt and shame for things you did or didn't do during your partner's depression. We all make mistakes and do things we regret. Rather than carrying that burden, learn from it and move on, seeking to do better in the future. As humans, we all screw up. Allow yourself to heal by letting it go. Partner-forgiveness and self-forgiveness will open the door to having a more rewarding, satisfying, and authentic relationship.

The Long and Winding Road

Depression can be a long and winding road, presenting many challenges and detours. Adrian began to realize that it wasn't helpful for him to view Margaret's depression as something that can be beaten and never comes back. He recognized that there were times when it got better, other times when it got worse, and moments when the couple felt completely overwhelmed and immobilized. Adrian started to focus on one day at a time. They met with psychiatrists and psychologists. Margaret tried various medications and psychological treatments, but nothing seemed to improve her depression. Adrian was able to provide hope, however. He encouraged Margaret to hang on a bit longer. They still had appointments. They still had options, and that realization got them through the darkest times.

The path involved in managing the difficulties and heartaches of a partner's depression may also be long and circuitous. You might find that you and your partner have tried different treatment approaches including psychotherapy, medication, or their combination, and are still wrestling with this disorder. Take it one step at a time.

Just as there are many ways to become depressed, there are, fortunately, many pathways out (see Chapter 3). A given treatment isn't a panacea for everyone. If your loved one has given a particular treatment enough time and effort—they received a sufficient "dose"—and still finds it unhelpful, don't lose hope; other options are likely available. Finding a treatment that works best will take time. Although it can be frustrating and demoralizing to keep trying new approaches, chances are good that you will land on one that will be a good match for your partner.

Research is starting to move toward more precision treatments that match techniques to vulnerabilities and specific treatments to certain individuals. We aren't quite there yet, but we are getting close. In the meantime, some trial and error may be needed to determine what will work best for your partner.

Finding Meaning through Suffering

The COVID-19 pandemic devastated the world from 2020–2023. Everyone was impacted by fear, uncertainty, lockdowns, and social distancing. There was so much pain and suffering. According to the World Health Organization, more than seven million people died directly from the virus. Frontline workers experienced symptoms of burnout and posttraumatic stress disorder. The economy was rocked. There were massive job losses and business closures. COVID-19 also contributed to a mental health crisis. People suffered from loneliness and social isolation. Anxiety and depression were at an all-time high, and many were dealing with grief and trauma.

Yet, during this crisis, people pulled together to support one another. In countries around the world people stood on balconies or doorsteps at 7 P.M. to bang pots and pans, clap, or cheer to honor exhausted frontline workers. Blue lights illuminated houses and landmarks around the globe to honor health care workers. In England, for example, the London Eye, Windsor Castle, and other landmarks shone in blue as a sign of respect for frontline workers. In Poland, Warsaw's Royal Castle and the Świętokrzyski Bridge were lit blue to show support for health care professionals. In the United States, the Space Needle, Pier 57, and other monuments in Seattle shone blue. In Canada, the CN Tower in Toronto, and other landmarks across the country, were lit up.

Acts of kindness were shown around the globe. People made masks for strangers, delivered food for those in need, and checked on isolated neighbors. Although grocery store shelves were emptied of toilet paper and other products due to panic buying, many people also rediscovered the simple things in life. They made bread and took up new hobbies and interests. There was also a collective reevaluation of what really matters in life—family, friends, health, time, and connection. We began to cherish these things even more. Many used this crisis to reprioritize their goals. We realized that we are not alone in our vulnerability. We learned that connection is critical. We looked inward and became more grateful for the simplicity of life. And we learned to slow down and savor what is important to us. Suffering can do that for us. It strips away the distractions and helps us understand what truly matters.

From 1942 to 1945, Austrian psychiatrist Viktor Frankl was imprisoned in Nazi concentration camps, including Auschwitz, where he lost his parents, brother, and pregnant wife. He witnessed the worst of humanity—unimaginable cruelty, dehumanization, torture, and starvation. In this suffering, Frankl observed that people who had a sense of purpose and meaning (even in the smallest of things) were more likely to survive. Frankl wrote a memoir titled *Man's Search for Meaning,* which became an international bestseller. He highlighted the fact that, even in the darkest moments, suffering can deepen us, and we can find meaning.

You may have experienced considerable psychological and emotional turmoil as you supported your loved one with depression. There were likely times when you felt emotionally and physically spent, confused, lonely, frustrated, and deep in despair. You may have wanted to give up. Your life may have been put on hold as you sacrificed your own needs and desires to care for your partner. These experiences, brutal as they may have been, can teach you lessons about who you are and what really matters to you.

TRY THIS: FINDING MEANING IN YOUR SUFFERING

Take a moment to reflect on your experiences. Is it possible for you to find meaning and purpose through them? Perhaps these sacrifices taught you more about what love is really about. For those who are married, wedding vows of "for better or for worse, for richer or for poorer, in sickness and in health" are often more poignant after 25 or 50 years of marriage because there have been opportunities to truly live these vows. Maybe this experience helped you discover what's most valuable and important to you. Consider the lessons your pain has taught you.

If you are open to learning what it can teach, the suffering you faced while supporting your partner can be transformative. These experiences invite us to grow and become stronger and more authentic versions of ourselves as individuals and as partners.

Maintaining Hope

Maintaining hope can be incredibly challenging, especially if your partner doesn't seem to be improving, the relationship remains shaky, or depression continues to return. Try to remind yourself that there are different pathways to recovery. It is often not a linear process, and setbacks don't mean failure. Try to challenge negative thoughts if they arise (see Chapters 6 and 12). Believing that "nothing will ever change" will only maintain hopelessness. Try to have realistic hope, or cautious optimism, recognizing that, although this is brutally hard, it won't last forever.

Think about times when you have overcome adversity in the past and try to use these experiences to propel you forward. Live in a way that is congruent with your values as an individual and as a couple (see Chapter 14). Celebrate the small victories. Ensure that you have a life outside of your partner's depression, staying connected to people and activities that matter to you (see Chapter 10). Try to set meaningful goals for yourself and your relationship, even if you need to start out small. Recognize that you have control over how you can manage this crisis. Finally, remember that if one approach doesn't work, others may.

Depression is difficult to manage, but it doesn't have to define who you are as individuals or as a couple. My hope is that the techniques and recommendations outlined in this book have given you the tools to help your partner overcome their depression, support you in coping with this difficulty, and improve your interactions as a couple. Wherever you are in the process of dealing with your partner's depression, I hope that you feel more armed and equipped with the strategies you've learned. Chances are good that you will eventually see light at the end of the tunnel. You can improve these odds by applying what you have learned in this book.

Resources

Here are some self-help books that you might find helpful for managing depression and various issues that couples confront. Also listed are websites to numerous agencies that provide information on dealing with mental health issues, including depression.

Recommended Self-Help Readings

Depression

Addis, M., & Martell, C. R. (2004). *Overcoming depression one step at a time: The new behavioral activation approach to getting your life back.* New Harbinger.

Bieling, P. J., & Antony, M. M. (2003). *Ending the depression cycle: A step-by-step guide for preventing relapse.* New Harbinger.

Clark, D. A. (2014). *The mood repair toolkit: Proven strategies to prevent the blues from turning into depression.* Guilford Press.

Greenberger, D., & Padesky, C. A. (2016). *Mind over mood: Change how you feel by changing the way you think* (2nd ed.). Guilford Press.

Hayes, S. C. (2025). *Get out of your mind and into your life: The new acceptance and commitment therapy.* New Harbinger.

Hershenberg, R. (2017). *A jump-start guide to overcoming low motivation, depression, or just feeling stuck.* New Harbinger.

Josefowitz, N., & Swallow, S. R. (2024). *The behavioral activation workbook for depression: Powerful strategies to boost your mood and build a better life.* New Harbinger.

Last, C. G. (2009). *When someone you love is bipolar: Help and support for you and your partner.* Guilford Press.

Miklowitz, D. J. (2024). *Living well with bipolar disorder: Practical strategies for improving your daily life.* Guilford Press.

Otto, M., & Smits, J. (2011). *Exercise for mood and anxiety: Proven strategies for overcoming depression and enhancing well-being.* Oxford University Press.

Paterson, R. J. (2016). *How to be miserable: 40 strategies you already use.* New Harbinger.

Rego, S., & Fader, S. (2018). *The 10-step depression relief workbook: A cognitive behavioral therapy approach.* Althea Press.

Strosahl, K. D., & Robinson, P. J. (2017). *The mindfulness and acceptance workbook for depression: Using acceptance and commitment therapy to move through depression and create a life worth living* (2nd ed.). New Harbinger.

Williams, M., Teasdale, J., Segal, Z., & Kabat-Zinn, J. (2025). *The mindful way through depression: Freeing yourself from chronic unhappiness* (2nd ed.). Guilford Press.

Wright, J. H., & McCray, L. W. (2012). *Breaking free from depression: Pathways to wellness.* Guilford Press.

Couple Issues

Becker, M. (2023). *Compassion for couples: Building skills of loving connection.* Guilford Press.

Christensen, A., Doss, B. D., & Jacobson, N. S. (2014). *Reconcilable differences: Rebuild your relationships by rediscovering the partner you love–without losing yourself.* Guilford Press.

Gottmann, J., & Silver, N. (2000). *The seven principles for making marriage work.* Harmony.

Nichols, M. P., & Straus, M. B. (2021). *The lost art of listening: How learning to listen can improve relationships* (3rd ed.). Guilford Press.

Snyder, D. K., Gordon, K. C., & Baucom, D. H. (2023). *Getting past the affair: A program to help you cope, heal, and move on—together or apart* (2nd ed.). Guilford Press.

Recommended Websites

Academy of Cognitive and Behavioral Therapies—Mainly an organization for professionals who practice cognitive-behavioral therapy; however, they do provide information on how CBT can help and a searchable list of providers who are certified in CBT.

www.academyofct.org

Anxiety and Depression Association of America (ADAA)—An organization providing online communities and other resources for anxiety and depression.

www.adaa.org

Association for Behavior and Cognitive Therapies—A professional organization that also provides evidence-based information for the public about treatments, fact sheets about different mental disorders, including depression, and recommended self-help books.

www.abct.org

Beck Institute—An organization mainly for professionals who practice CBT; however, they also provide information about CBT for the general public.

https://beckinstitute.org/cbt-resources

Befrienders Worldwide—A network of emotional-support centres in many countries that helps people in distress, including those with depression and suicidal thoughts.

https://befrienders.org

Beyond Blue (Australia)—A globally renowned mental health research not-for-profit agency that focuses on anxiety, depression & suicide prevention.

www.beyondblue.org.au/mental-health

Black Dog Institute (Australia)—An organization providing digital tools, apps, fact sheets and other research for managing depression, anxiety, bipolar disorder, and suicidal thinking.

www.blackdoginstitute.org.au

Canadian Mental Health Association—A national charity promoting mental health and supporting people recovering from mental illness, with branches across the country. Includes information and fact sheets on various mental health problems.

www.cmha.ca

Centre for Clinical Interventions (Australia)—A clinical psychology organization that provides self-help resources for mental health problems.

www.cci.health.wa.gov.au/Resources/Looking-After-Yourself

Depression and Bipolar Support Alliance—An organization that provides peer-led support, tools and resources for individuals dealing with depression and bipolar disorder.

www.dbsalliance.org

European Alliance Against Depression (EAAD)—A nonprofit association that speaks up for individuals impacted by depression and has resources geared to depression and suicide prevention. The iFightDepression tool is a free, web-based program designed to help individuals with mild to moderate depression using principles of cognitive-behavioral therapy.

www.eaad.net

https://tool.ifightdepression.com/en-ad/login

Mood Disorders Society of Canada—An organization that provides information about depression and available treatments.

www.mdsc.ca

National Alliance on Mental Illness—An organization providing information about mental health disorders (including depressive disorders) and treatments; also has podcasts and webinars.

www.nami.org

National Health Service (United Kingdom)—An organization that provides information about depression and other mental health conditions and self-help tools.

www.nhs.uk/mental-health

National Institute of Mental Health—The lead federal agency in the United States for research on mental disorders, including depression. Provides free, evidence-based information about depression.

www.nimh.nih.gov/health/find-help

World Health Organization (WHO)—The United Nations health agency that provides facts and guidance on depression and mental health globally.

www.who.int/health-topics/depression

Bibliography

Chapter 1. Understanding the Experience of Depression

American Psychiatric Association. (2022). *Diagnostic and statistical manual of mental disorders* (5th ed., text rev.). Author.

Cassidy, J., Jones, J. D., & Shaver, P. R. (2013). Contributions of attachment theory and research: A framework for future research, translation, and policy. *Developmental Psychopathology, 25,* 1415–1434.

Cuijpers, P., Miguel, C., Harrer, M., Plessen, C. Y., Ciharova, M., Ebert, D., & Karyotaki, E. (2023). Cognitive behavior therapy vs. control conditions, other psychotherapies, pharmacotherapies and combined treatment for depression: A comprehensive meta-analysis including 409 trials with 52,702 patients. *World Psychiatry, 22,* 105–115.

Dell'Osso, B., Cafaro, R., & Ketter, T. A. (2021). Has bipolar disorder become a predominantly female gender related condition? Analysis of recently published large sample studies. *International Journal of Bipolar Disorder, 9*(1), 3.

Dozois, D. J. A., & Beck, A. T. (2023). Negative thinking in depression: Cognitive products and schema structures. In D. J. A. Dozois & K. S. Dobson (Eds.), *Treatment of psychosocial risk factors in depression* (pp. 207–232). American Psychological Association.

Dozois, D. J. A., & Dobson, K. S. (Eds.). (2023). *Treatment of psychosocial risk factors in depression.* American Psychological Association.

Dozois, D. J. A., Wilde, J. L., & Dobson, K. S. (2020). Depressive disorders. In M. M. Antony & D. H. Barlow (Eds.), *Handbook of assessment and treatment planning for psychological disorders* (3rd ed., pp. 335–378). Guilford Press.

Hasin, D. S., Sarvet, A. L., Meyers, J. L., Saha, T. D., Ruan, W. J., Stohl, M., & Grant, B. F. (2018). Epidemiology of adult DSM-5 major depressive disorder and its specifiers in the United States. *JAMA Psychiatry, 75*(4), 336–346.

Kendler, K. S. (2019). From many to one to many: The search for causes of psychiatric illness. *JAMA Psychiatry, 76,* 1085–1091.

Lim, G. Y., Tam, W. W., Lu, Y., Ho, C. S., Zhang, M. W., & Ho, R. C. (2018). Prevalence of depression in the community from 30 countries between 1994 and 2014. *Scientific Reports, 8,* 2861.

Rehman, U. S., Gollan, J., & Mortimer, A. R. (2008). The marital context of depression: Research, limitations, and new directions. *Clinical Psychology Review, 28*(2), 179–198.

Whisman, M. A., Sbarra, D. A., & Beach, S. R. H. (2021). Intimate relationships and depression: Searching for causation in the sea of association. *Annual Review of Clinical Psychology, 7*(17), 233–258.

World Health Organization. (2022). *ICD-11: International classification of diseases* (11th rev.). *https://icd.who.int*

Chapter 2. Supporting Your Partner Effectively

Bowlby, J. (1980). *Attachment and loss: Loss—Sadness and depression* (vol. 3, International Psycho-Analytical Library Series No. 109). Hogarth Press.

Bowlby, J. (1988). *A secure base: Parent-child attachment and healthy human development.* Basic Books.

Brooks, D. (2023). *How to know a person: The art of seeing others deeply and being deeply seen* (pp. 113–114). Random House.

Choi, K. W., Stein, M. B., Nishimi, K. M., Ge, T., Coleman, J. R. I., Chen, C.-Y., Ratanatharathorn, A., Zheutlin, A. B., Dunn, E. C., 23andMe Research Team, Major Depressive Disorder Working Group of the Psychiatric Genomics Consortium, Breen, G., Koenen, K. C., & Smoller, J. W. (2020). An exposure-wide and Mendelian randomization approach to identifying modifiable factors for the prevention of depression. *American Journal of Psychiatry, 177,* 944–954.

Feeney, B. C., & Collins, N. L. (2018). Social support in close relationships. In A. L. Vangelisti & D. Perlman (Eds.), *The Cambridge handbook of personal relationships* (2nd ed., pp. 282–296). Cambridge University Press.

Gariépy, G., Honkaniemi, H., & Quesnel-Vallée, A. (2016). Social support and protection from depression: Systematic review of current findings in Western countries. *British Journal of Psychiatry, 209*(4), 284–293.

Givertz, M., & Safford, S. (2011). Longitudinal impact of communication patterns on romantic attachment and symptoms of depression. *Current Psychology: A Journal for Diverse Perspectives on Diverse Psychological Issues, 30*(2), 148–172.

Holt-Lunstad, J., Smith, T. B., Baker, M., Harris, T., & Stephenson, D. (2015). Loneliness and social isolation as risk factors for mortality: A meta-analytic review. *Perspectives on Psychological Science, 10,* 227–237.

Holt-Lunstad, J., Smith, T. B., & Layton, J. B. (2010). Social relationships and mortality risk: A meta-analytic review. *PLOS Medicine, 7,* e1000316.

Kammrath, L. (2024, July). *Hard to be a supporter. Hard to think of what to say. Am I saying the right thing? Selection rules.* Paper presented at the International Association of Relationships Research conference, Boston, MA.

LaBuda, J. E., & Gere, J. (2023). A meta-analytic review of accuracy and bias in romantic partner perceptions. *Psychological Bulletin, 149*(9–10), 580–610.

MacKinney, L., Yamamoto, E., Ji, L., Ard, T., Haga, S., Zhao, Y., & Kammrath, L. (2024, July). *Disentangling the elements of emotional support: Connect versus cope* [Poster presentation]. International Association of Relationships Research conference, Boston, MA.

Marroquín B. (2011). Interpersonal emotion regulation as a mechanism of social support in depression. *Clinical Psychology Review, 31*(8), 1276–1290.

McLeod, S., Berry, K., Hodgson, C., & Wearden, A. (2020). Attachment and social support in romantic dyads: A systematic review. *Journal of Clinical Psychology, 76*(1), 59–101.

Miller, W. R., & Rollnick, S. (2023). *Motivational interviewing: Helping people change* (4th ed.). Guilford Press.

Muschetto, T., & Siegel, J. T. (2019). Attribution theory and support for individuals with depression: The impact of controllability, stability, and interpersonal relationship. *Stigma and Health, 4,* 126–135.

Nichols, M. P., & Straus, M. B. (2021). *The lost art of listening: How learning to listen can improve relationships* (3rd. ed.). Guilford Press.

Rogers, C. R. (1959). A theory of therapy, personality, and interpersonal relationships: As developed in the client-centered framework. In S. Koch (Ed.), *Psychology: A study of a science—Formulations of the person and the social context* (Vol. 3, pp. 184–256). McGraw Hill.

Rogers, C. R. (1986). Carl Rogers on the development of the person-centered approach. *Person-Centered Review, 1*(3), 257–259.

Solomon, D. A., Keller, M. B., Leon, A. C., Mueller, T. I., Lavori, P. W., Shea, M. T., Coryell, W., Warshaw, M., Turvey, C., Maser, J. D., & Endicott, J. (2000). Multiple recurrences of major depressive disorder. *American Journal of Psychiatry, 157*(2), 229–233.

Wang, J., Mann, F., Lloyd-Evans, B., Ma, R., & Johnson, S. (2018). Associations between loneliness and perceived social support and outcomes of mental health problems: A systematic review. *BMC Psychiatry, 18*(5).

Yao, E., & Siegel, J. T. (2021). The influence of perceptions of intentionality and controllability on perceived responsibility: Applying attribution theory to people's responses to social transgression in the COVID-19 pandemic. *Motivation Science, 7*(2), 199–206.

Yeo, G., Lansford, J. E., & Rudolph, K. D. (2025). How does perceived social support relate to human thriving? A systematic review with meta-analyses. *Psychological Bulletin, 151*(9), 1089–1124.

Zell, E., & Stockus, C. A. (2025). Social support and psychological adjustment: A quantitative synthesis of 60 meta-analyses. *American Psychologist, 80*(1), 33–46.

Chapter 3. Becoming Informed about Treatments That Help

American Psychological Association. (2019). Clinical practice guidelines for the treatment of depression across three age cohorts. *www.apa.org/depression-guideline/guideline.pdf*

Beck, A. T., & Dozois, D. J. A. (2011). Cognitive therapy: Current status and future directions. *Annual Review of Medicine, 62,* 397–409.

Beck, A. T., Rush, A. J., Shaw, B. F., Emery, G., DeRubeis, R. J., & Hollon, S. D. (2024). *Cognitive therapy of depression* (2nd ed.). Guilford Press.

Cuijpers, P., Noma, H., Karyotaki, E., Vinkers, C. H., Cipriani, A., & Furukawa, T. A. (2020). A network meta-analysis of the effects of psychotherapies, pharmacotherapies and their combination in the treatment of adult depression. *World Psychiatry, 19*(1), 92–107.

DeRubeis, R. J., Hollon, S. D., Amsterdam, J. D, Shelton, R. C., Young, P. R., Salomon, R. M., O'Reardon, J. P., Lovett, M. L., Gladis, M. M , Brown, L. L., & Gallop, R. (2005). Cognitive therapy vs. medications in the treatment of moderate to severe depression. *Archives of General Psychiatry, 62*(4), 409–416.

DeRubeis, R. J., Keefe, J. R., & Beck, A. T. (2019). Cognitive therapy. In K. S. Dobson & D. J. A. Dozois (Eds.), *Handbook of cognitive-behavioral therapies* (4th ed., pp. 218–248). Guilford Press.

Dobson, D., & Dobson, K. S. (2017). *Evidence-based practice of cognitive-behavioral therapy* (2nd ed.). Guilford Press.

Dozois, D. J. A., Dobson, K. S., & Rnic, K. (2019). Historical and philosophical bases of the cognitive-behavioral therapies. In K. S. Dobson & D. J. A. Dozois (Eds.), *Handbook of cognitive-behavioral therapies* (4th ed., pp. 3–31). Guilford Press.

Fregni, F., El-Hagrassy, M. M., Pacheco-Barrios, K., Carvalho, S., Leite, J., Simis, M., Brunelin, J., Nakamura-Palacios, E. M., Marangolo, P., Venkatasubramanian, G., San-Juan, D., Caumo, W., Bikson, M., Brunoni, A. R., & Neuromodulation Center Working Group. (2021). Evidence-based guidelines and secondary meta-analysis for the use of transcranial direct current stimulation in neurological and psychiatric disorders. *International Journal of Neuropsychopharmacology, 24*(4), 256–313.

Guideline Development Panel for the Treatment of Depressive Disorders. (2022). Summary of the clinical practice guideline for the treatment of depression across three age cohorts. *American Psychologist, 77*(6), 770–780.

Hollon, S. D., Andrews, P. W., Keller, M. C., Singla, D. R., Maslej, M. M., & Mulsant, B. H. (2021). Combining psychotherapy and medications: It's all about the squids and the sea bass (at least for nonpsychotic patients). In M. Barkham, W. Lutz, & L. G. Castonguay (Eds.), *Bergin and Garfield's handbook of psychotherapy and behavior change: 50th anniversary edition* (7th ed., pp. 705–738). Wiley.

Hollon, S. D., DeRubeis, R. J., Shelton, R. C., Amsterdam, J. D., Salomon, R. M., O'Reardon, J. P., Lovett, M. L., Young, P. R., Haman, K. L., Freeman, B. B., & Gallop, R. (2005). Prevention of relapse following cognitive therapy vs. medications in moderate to severe depression. *Archives of General Psychiatry, 62*(4), 417–422.

Lam, C., & Chung, M. H. (2021). A meta-analysis of the effect of interpersonal and social rhythm therapy on symptom and functioning improvement in patients with bipolar disorders. *Applied Research Quality Life, 16,* 153–165.

Lam, D. H., Jones, S. H., & Hayward, P. (2010). *Cognitive therapy for bipolar disorder: A therapist's guide to concepts, methods and practice.* Wiley.

Lam, R. W., Kennedy, S. H., Adams, C., Bahji, A., Beaulieu, S., Bhat, V., Blier, P., Blumberger, D. M., Brietzke, E., Chakrabarty, T., Do, A., Frey, B. N., Giacobbe, P., Gratzer, D., Grigoriadis, S., Habert, J., Husain, M. I., Ismail, Z., McGirr, A., & McIntyre, R. S. (2024). Canadian Network for Mood and Anxiety Treatments (CANMAT) 2023 Update on clinical guidelines for management of major depressive disorder in adults. *Canadian Journal of Psychiatry, 69*(9), 641–687.

Martell, C. R., Dimidjian, S., & Herman-Dunn, R. (2022). *Behavioral activation for depression: A clinician's guide* (2nd ed.). Guilford Press.

Martell, C. R., & Puspitasari, A. J. (2023). Cognitive and behavioral avoidance. In

D. J. A. Dozois & K. S. Dobson (Eds.), *Treatment of psychosocial risk factors in depression* (pp. 359–381). American Psychological Association.

Miklowitz, D. J., & Chung, B. (2016). Family-focused therapy for bipolar disorder: Reflections on 30 years of research. *Family Process, 55*(3), 483–499.

Miklowitz, D. J., Efthimiou, O., Furukawa, T. A., Scott, J., McLaren, R., Geddes, J. R., & Cipriani, A. (2021). Adjunctive psychotherapy for bipolar disorder: A systematic review and component network meta-analysis. *JAMA Psychiatry, 78*(2), 141–150.

Miklowitz, D. J., Otto, M. W., Frank, E., Reilly-Harrington, N. A., Wisniewski, S. R., Kogan, J. N., Nierenberg, A. A., Calabrese, J. R., Marangell, L. B., Gyulai, L., Araga. M., Gonzalez, J. M., Shirley, E. R., Thase. M. E., & Sachs, G. S. (2007). Psychosocial treatments for bipolar depression: A 1-year randomized trial from the systematic treatment enhancement program. *Archives of General Psychiatry, 64*(4), 419–426.

Miller, W. R., & Rollnick, S. (2023). *Motivational interviewing: Helping people change* (4th ed.). Guilford Press.

Moncrieff, J., Cooper, R. E., Stockmann, T., Amendola, S., Hengartner, M. P., & Horowitz, M. A. (2023). The serotonin theory of depression: A systematic umbrella review of the evidence. *Molecular Psychiatry, 28*, 3243–3256.

National Institute for Clinical Excellence. (2018). Depression in adults: Depression: Treatment and management (draft guideline for second consultation). Retrieved July 20, 2018, from *www.nice.org.uk/guidance/gid-cgwave0725/documents/short-version-of-draft-guideline*

Parikh, S. V., Kcomt, A., Fonseka, T. M., Pong, J. T. (Eds). (2018). *The CHOICE–D patient and family guide to depression treatment.* Mood Disorders Association of Ontario.

Perricone, A., & Ahn, W. (2023). Reasons for the belief that psychotherapy is less effective for biologically attributed mental disorders. *Cognitive Therapy and Research, 48(4), 599609.*

Shafran, R., Egan, S. J., de Valle, M., Davey, E., Carlbring, P., Creswell, C., & Wade, T. D. (2024). A guide for self-help guides: best practice implementation. *Cognitive Behaviour Therapy, 53*(5), 561–575.

Watson, L. M., & Beshai, S. (2021). Causal explanations of depression on perceptions of and likelihood to choose cognitive behavioural therapy and antidepressant medications as depression treatments. *Psychology and Psychotherapy: Theory, Research and Practice, 94*(2), 201–216.

Whitaker, R. (2015). *Anatomy of an epidemic: Magic bullets, psychiatric drugs, and the astonishing rise of mental illness in America.* Random House.

Chapter 4. Encouraging Treatment

Alves, S., Martins, A., Fonseca, A., Canavarro, M. C., & Pereira, M. (2018). Preventing and treating women's postpartum depression: A qualitative systematic review on partner-inclusive interventions. *Journal of Child and Family Studies, 27*(1), 1–25.

Baker-Russell, L. (2015). *Adding insult to injury: The implications of partner-regulation behaviors depend on partners' depressive symptoms* (Order No. AAI3637943). Available from APA PsycInfo®. (1709218931; 2015-99161-039). Retrieved from *www.lib.*

uwo.ca/cgi-bin/ezpauthn.cgi?url=http://search.proquest.com/dissertations-theses/adding-insult-injury-implications-partner/docview/1709218931/se-2

Collins, K. A., Westra, H. A., Dozois, D. J. A., & Burns, D. D. (2004). Gaps in accessing treatment for anxiety and depression: Challenges for the delivery of care. *Clinical Psychology Review, 24*(5), 583–616.

Dobson, K. S., Hollon, S. D., Dimidjian, S., Schmaling, K. B., Kohlenberg, R. J., Gallop, R. J., Rizvi, S. L., Gollan, J. K., Dunner, D. L., & Jacobson, N. S. (2008). Randomized trial of behavioral activation, cognitive therapy, and antidepressant medication in the prevention of relapse and recurrence in major depression. *Journal of Consulting and Clinical Psychology, 76*(3), 468–477.

Dozois, D. J. A., & Mental Health Research Canada (2021). Anxiety and depression in Canada during the COVID-19 pandemic: A national survey. *Canadian Psychology, 62,* 136–142.

Dozois, D. J. A., & Westra, H. A. (2005). The development of the Anxiety Change Expectancy Scale (ACES) and validation in college, community, and clinical samples. *Behaviour Research and Therapy, 43,* 1655–1672.

Dozois, D. J. A., Wilde, J. L., & Dobson, K. S. (2020). Depressive disorders. In M. M. Antony & D. H. Barlow (Eds.), *Handbook of assessment and treatment planning for psychological disorders* (3rd ed., pp. 335–378). Guilford Press.

Falconier, M. K., & Kuhn, R. (2019). Dyadic coping in couples: A conceptual integration and a review of the empirical literature. *Frontiers in Psychology, 10,* Article 571.

Goodwin, R. D., Dierker, L. C., Wu, M. Galea, S., Hoven, C. W., & Weinberger, A. H. (2022). Trends in U.S. depression prevalence from 2015 to 2020: The widening treatment gap. *American Journal of Preventive Medicine, 63*(5), 726–733.

Hansen, M. C., Fuentes, D., & Aranda, M. P. (2018). Re-engagement into care: The role of social support on service use for recurrent episodes of mental health distress among primary care patients. *Journal of Behavioral Health Services and Research, 45,* 90–104.

Hershenberg, R., Mavandadi, S., Klaus, J. R., Oslin, D. W., & Sayers, S. L. (2014). Veteran preferences for romantic partner involvement in depression treatment. *General Hospital Psychiatry, 36*(6), 757–759.

Krebs, P., Norcross, J. C., Nicholson, J. M., & Prochaska, J. O. (2018). Stages of change and psychotherapy outcomes: A review and meta-analysis. *Journal of Clinical Psychology, 74*(11), 1964–1979.

Leuchtmann, L., & Bodenmann, G. (2017). Interpersonal view on physical illnesses and mental disorders: A systemic-transactional understanding of disorders. *Swiss Archives of Neurology, Psychiatry and Psychotherapy, 168*(6), 170–174.

Misri, S., Kostaras, X., Fox, D., & Kostaras, D. (2000). The impact of partner support in the treatment of postpartum depression. *Canadian Journal of Psychiatry, 45*(6), 554–558.

Neal, R. L., & Radomsky, A. S. (2020). What do you really need? Self-and partner-reported intervention preferences within cognitive behavioural therapy for reassurance seeking behaviour. *Behavioural and Cognitive Psychotherapy, 48*(1), 25–37.

Pratt, L. A., & Brody, D. J. (2014). Depression in the U.S. household population, 2009–2012. *NCHS Data Brief* (172), 1–8.

Siegel, J. T., Ellis, B., Riazi, G., Brafford, A., Guldner, G., & Wells, J. C. (2024). The paradox of the resident experiencing depression: Higher depression, less favorable help-seeking outcome expectations, and lower help-seeking intentions. *Social Science and Medicine, 344.*

Westra, H. A., & Dozois, D. J. A. (2008). Integrating motivational interviewing into the treatment of anxiety. In H. Arkowitz, H. A. Westra, W. R. Miller, & S. Rollnick (Eds.), *Motivational interviewing in the treatment of psychological problems* (pp. 26–56). Guilford Press.

Chapter 5. Helping Your Partner Engage in Antidepressant Behavior

Josefowitz, N., & Swallow, S. R. (2024). *The behavioral activation workbook for depression: Powerful strategies to boost your mood and build a better life.* New Harbinger.

Leahy, R. L., Clark, D. A., & Dozois, D. J. A. (2023). Theory of cognitive-behavioral therapy. In H. Crisp & G. O. Gabbard (Eds.), D. Sudak & S. Bhatt-Mackin (Section Ed.), *Gabbard's textbook of psychotherapeutic treatments* (2nd ed., pp. 151–167). American Psychiatric Press.

Martell, C. R., Dimidjian, S., & Herman-Dunn, R. (2022). *Behavioral activation for depression: A clinician's guide* (2nd ed.). Guilford Press.

Martell, C. R., & Puspitasari, A. J. (2023). Cognitive and behavioral avoidance. In D. J. A. Dozois & K. S. Dobson (Eds.), *Treatment of psychosocial risk factors in depression* (pp. 359–381). American Psychological Association.

Chapter 6. Helping Your Partner Change Negative Thinking

Beck, A. T., & Dozois, D. J. A. (2014). Cognitive theory and therapy: Past, present and future. In S. Bloch, S. A. Green, & J. Holmes (Eds.), *Psychiatry—Past, present and prospect* (pp. 366–382). Oxford University Press.

Dozois, D. J. A., & Beck, A. T. (2008). Cognitive schemas, beliefs and assumptions. In K. S. Dobson & D. J. A. Dozois (Eds.), *Risk factors in depression* (pp. 121–143). Elsevier/Academic Press.

Dozois, D. J. A., & Beck, A. T. (2023). Negative thinking in depression: Cognitive products and schema structures. In D. J. A. Dozois & K. S. Dobson (Eds.), *Treatment of psychosocial risk factors in depression* (pp. 207–232). American Psychological Association.

Greenberger, D., & Padesky, C. A. (2016). *Mind over mood: Change how you feel by changing the way you think* (2nd ed.). Guilford Press.

Chapter 7. Being Aware of Warning Signs and Managing Expectations

Alnefeesi, Y., Chen-Li, D., Krane, E., Jawad, M. Y., Rodrigues, N. B., Ceban, F., Di Vincenzo, J. D., Meshkat, S., Ho, R. C. M., Gill, H., Teopiz, K. M., Cao, B., Lee, Y., McIntyre, R. S., & Rosenblat, J. D. (2022). Real-world effectiveness of ketamine in treatment-resistant depression: A systematic review & meta-analysis. *Journal of Psychiatric Research, 151,* 693–709.

American Psychiatric Association. (2022). *Diagnostic and statistical manual of mental disorders* (5th ed., text rev.). Author.

Canadian Mental Health Association. (n.d.). *Safety plans to prevent suicide: A suicide prevention toolkit.* Retrieved February 26, 2025, from *www.suicideinfo.ca/wp-content/uploads/2019/09/SafetyPlan_Toolkit_0919_web.pdf*

Conley, A. A., Norwood, A. E. Q., Hatvany, T. C., Griffith, J. D., & Barber, K. E. (2021). Efficacy of ketamine for major depressive episodes at 2, 4, and 6-weeks post-treatment: A meta-analysis. *Psychopharmacology, 238*(7), 1737–1752.

Joiner, T. E. (2005). *Why people die by suicide.* Harvard University Press.

Kessler, R. C., de Jonge, P., Shahly, V., van Loo, H. M., Wang, P. S.-E., & Wilcox, M. A. (2014). Epidemiology of depression. In I. H. Gotlib & C. L. Hammen (Eds.), *Handbook of depression* (3rd ed., pp. 7–24). Guilford Press.

Klein, D. N., & Allmann, A. E. S. (2014). Course of depression: Persistence and recurrence. In I. H. Gotlib & C. L. Hammen (Eds.), *Handbook of depression* (3rd ed., pp. 64–83). Guilford Press.

Klonsky, E. D., Pachkowski, M. C., Shahnaz, A., & May, A. M. (2021). The three-step theory of suicide: Description, evidence, and some useful points of clarification. *Preventive Medicine, 152*(Pt 1), 106549.

Knapp, S. (2023). The essentials of creating effective safety planning-type interventions for suicidal patients. *Practice Innovations, 8*(2), 131–140.

May, A. M., & Klonsky, E. D. (2013). Assessing motivations for suicide attempts: Development and psychometric properties of the inventory of motivations for suicide attempts. *Suicide and Life-Threatening Behavior, 43*(5), 532–546.

May, A. M., Pachkowski, M. C., & Klonsky, E. D. (2020). Motivations for suicide: Converging evidence from clinical and community samples. *Journal of Psychiatric Research, 123,* 171–177.

Solomon, D. A., Keller, M. B., Leon, A. C., Mueller, T. I., Lavori, P. W., Shea, M. T., Coryell, W., Warshaw, M., Turvey, C., Maser, J. D., & Endicott, J. (2000). Multiple recurrences of major depressive disorder. *American Journal of Psychiatry, 157,* 229–233.

U.S. Department of Health and Human Services. (2024, April). *National strategy for suicide prevention.* Author.

World Health Organization. (2024, August). *Suicide. www.who.int/news-room/fact-sheets/detail/suicide*

Chapter 8. Making Sense of Your Feelings and Tending to Your Needs

Benazon, N. R., & Coyne, J. C. (2000). Living with a depressed spouse. *Journal of Family Psychology, 14*(1), 71–79.

Falconier, M. K., & Kuhn, R. (2019). Dyadic coping in couples: A conceptual integration and a review of the empirical literature. *Frontiers in Psychology, 10,* Article 571.

Holt-Lunstad, J. (2024). Social connection as a critical factor for mental and physical health: Evidence, trends, challenges, and future implications. *World Psychiatry, 23*(3), 312–332.

Kiecolt-Glaser, J. K., & Wilson, S. J. (2017). Lovesick: How couples' relationships influence health. *Annual Review of Clinical Psychology, 13,* 421–443.

Nall, R. (2024, August). *Handling a breakup with someone with depression. www.healthline.com/health/depression/relationships*

Perlick, D. A., Berk, L., Kaczynski, R., Gonzalez, J., Link, B., Dixon, L., Grier, S., & Miklowitz, D. J. (2016). Caregiver burden as a predictor of depression among family and friends who provide care for persons with bipolar disorder. *Bipolar Disorders, 18*(2), 183–191.

Priestley, J., & McPherson, S. (2016). Experiences of adults providing care to a partner or relative with depression: A meta-ethnographic synthesis. *Journal of Affective Disorders, 192,* 41–49.

Randall, A. K., & Bodenmann, G. (2017). Stress and its associations with relationship satisfaction. *Current Opinion in Psychology, 13,* 96–106.

Sharabi, L. L., Delaney, A. L., & Knobloch, L. K. (2016). In their own words: How clinical depression affects romantic relationships. *Journal of Social and Personal Relationships, 33*(4), 421–448.

Skundberg-Kletthagen, H., Wangensteen, S., Hall-Lord, M. L., & Hedelin, B. (2014). Relatives of patients with depression: Experiences of everyday life. *Scandinavian Journal of Caring Sciences, 28*(3), 564–571.

Stjernswärd, S., & Östman, M. (2008). Whose life am I living? Relatives living in the shadow of depression. *International Journal of Social Psychiatry, 54*(4), 358–369.

Swinkels, J., van Tilburg, T., Verbakel, E., & Broese van Groenou, M. (2019). Explaining the gender gap in the caregiving burden of partner caregivers. *Journals of Gerontology: Series B, 74*(2), 309–317.

Chapter 9. Understanding Your Responsibility

Gaiman, N. (2008). *The graveyard book.* HarperCollins.

Halgin, R. P., & Lovejoy, D. W. (1991). An integrative approach to treating the partner of a depressed person. *Psychotherapy: Theory, Research, Practice, Training, 28*(2), 251–258.

Priestley, J., & McPherson, S. (2016). Experiences of adults providing care to a partner or relative with depression: A meta-ethnographic synthesis. *Journal of Affective Disorders, 192,* 41–49.

Zayfert, C., & DeVina, J. C. (2011). *When someone you love suffers from posttraumatic stress: What to expect and what you can do.* Guilford Press.

Chapter 10. Putting Structure and Routine Back into Your Life

Baranwal, N., Yu, P. K., & Siegel, N. S. (2023). Sleep physiology, pathophysiology, and sleep hygiene. *Progress in Cardiovascular Diseases, 77,* 59–69.

Carney, C. E., Edinger, J. D., Kuchibhatla, M., Lachowski, A. M., Bogouslavsky, O., Krystal, A. D., & Shapiro, C. M. (2017). Cognitive behavioral insomnia therapy for those with insomnia and depression: A randomized controlled clinical trial. *Sleep,* 40(4), zsx019.

Carney, C. E., & Mamber, R. (2013). *Goodnight mind: Turn off your noisy thoughts and get a good night's sleep.* New Harbinger.

Cheung, J. M. Y., Jarrin, D. C., Ballot, O., Bharwani, A. A., & Morin, C. M. (2019). A systematic review of cognitive behavioral therapy for insomnia implemented in primary care and community settings. *Sleep Medicine Reviews, 44,* 23–36.

De Pasquale, C., El Kazzi, M., Sutherland, K., Shriane, A. E., Vincent, G. E., Cistulli, P. A., & Bin, Y. S. (2024). Sleep hygiene—What do we mean? A bibliographic review. *Sleep Medicine Reviews, 75,* 101930.

Diener, E., Heintzelman, S. J., Kushlev, K., Tay, L., Wirtz, D., Lutes, L. D., & Oishi, S. (2017). Findings all psychologists should know from the new science on subjective well-being. *Canadian Psychology / Psychologie canadienne, 58*(2), 87–104.

Dinu, M., Pagliai, G., Casini, A., & Sofi, F. (2018). Mediterranean diet and multiple health outcomes: An umbrella review of meta-analyses of observational studies and randomised trials. *European Journal of Clinical Nutrition, 72*(1), 30–43.

Dozois, D. J. A. (2018). Presidential address—Not the years in your life, but the life in your years: Lessons from Canadian psychology on living fully. *Canadian Psychology, 59,* 107–119.

Firth, J., Marx, W., Dash, S., Carney, R., Teasdale, S. B., Solmi, M., Stubbs, B., Schuch, F. B., Carvalho, A. F., Jacka, F., & Sarris, J. (2019). The effects of dietary improvement on symptoms of depression and anxiety: A meta-analysis of randomized controlled trials. *Psychosomatic Medicine, 81*(3), 265–280.

Holt-Lunstad, J. (2024). Social connection as a critical factor for mental and physical health: Evidence, trends, challenges, and future implications. *World Psychiatry, 23*(3), 312–332.

Holt-Lunstad, J., Smith, T. B., Baker, M., Harris, T., & Stephenson, D. (2015). Loneliness and social isolation as risk factors for mortality: A meta-analytic review. *Perspectives on Psychological Science, 10*(2), 227–237.

Mead, R. (2018, January 26). What Britain's "Minister of Loneliness" says about Brexit and the legacy of Jo Cox. *New Yorker. www.newyorker.com/culture/cultural-comment/britain-minister-of-loneliness-brexit-jo-cox*

Statistics Canada. (2021). *Canadian social survey: Loneliness in Canada. https://www150.statcan.gc.ca/n1/en/daily-quotidien/211124/dq211124e-eng.pdf?st=gR2vQlsg*

U.S. Department of Health and Human Services. (2023). *Our epidemic of loneliness and isolation: The U.S. Surgeon General's advisory on the healing effects of social connection and community.* U.S. Department of Health and Human Services. *www.hhs.gov/sites/default/files/surgeon-general-social-connection-advisory.pdf*

White, R. L., Vella, S., Biddle, S., Sutcliffe, J., Guagliano, J. M., Uddin, R., Burgin, A., Apostolopoulos, M., Nguyen, T., Young, C., Taylor, N., Lilley, S., & Teychenne, M. (2024). Physical activity and mental health: A systematic review and best-evidence synthesis of mediation and moderation studies. *International Journal of Behavioral Nutrition and Physical Activity, 21*(134).

Zaccaro, A., Piarulli, A., Laurino, M., Garbella, E., Menicucci, D., Neri, B., & Gemignani, A. (2018). How breath-control can change your life: a systematic review on psycho-physiological correlates of slow breathing. *Frontiers in Human Neuroscience, 12,* 353.

Chapter 11. Common Pitfalls and Thorny Issues

Barbato, A., & D'Avanzo, B. (2020). The findings of a Cochrane meta-analysis of couple therapy in adult depression: Implications for research and clinical practice. *Family Process 59,* 361–375.

Beach, S. R. H., Sandeen, E. E., & O'Leary, K. D. (1990). *Depression in marriage: A model for etiology and treatment.* Guilford Press.

Davila, J., Stroud, C. B., & Starr, L. R. (2014). Depression in couples and families. In I. H. Gotlib & C. L. Hammen (Eds.), *Handbook of depression* (3rd ed., pp. 410–428). Guilford Press.

Epstein, N. B., & Falconier, M. K. (2024). *Treatment plans and interventions in couple therapy: A cognitive-behavioral approach.* Guilford Press.

Evraire, L. E., & Dozois, D. J. A. (2011). An integrative model of excessive reassurance seeking and negative feedback seeking in the development and maintenance of depression. *Clinical Psychology Review, 31,* 1291–1303.

Evraire, L. E., & Dozois, D. J. A. (2014). If it be love indeed tell me how much: Early core beliefs associated with excessive reassurance seeking in depression. *Canadian Journal of Behavioural Science, 46,* 1–8.

Evraire, L. E., Dozois, D. J. A., & Wilde, J. (2022). The contribution of attachment styles and reassurance seeking to trust in romantic couples. *Europe's Journal of Psychology, 18,* 19–39.

Evraire, L. E., Ludmer, J. A., & Dozois, D. J. A. (2014). The influence of priming attachment styles on excessive reassurance seeking and negative feedback seeking in depression. *Journal of Social and Clinical Psychology, 33,* 295–318.

Gonçalves, W. S., Gherman, B. R., Abdo, C. H. N., Coutinho, E. S. F., Nardi, A. E., & Appolinario, J. C. (2023). Prevalence of sexual dysfunction in depressive and persistent depressive disorders: A systematic review and meta-analysis. *International Journal of Impotence Research, 35*(4), 340–349.

Laumann, E. O., Paik, A., & Rosen, R. C. (1999). Sexual dysfunction in the United States: Prevalence and predictors. *JAMA, 281*(6), 537–544.

Neal, R. L., & Radomsky, A. S. (2020). What do you really need? Self- and partner-reported intervention preferences within cognitive behavioural therapy for reassurance seeking behaviour. *Behavioural and Cognitive Psychotherapy, 48*(1), 25–37.

Rnic, K., Santee, A. C., Hoffmeister, J., Liu, H., Chang, K. K., Chen, R. X., Neufeld, R. W. J., Machado, D. A., Starr, L. R., Dozois, D. J. A., & LeMoult, J. (2023). The vicious cycle of psychopathology and stressful life events: A meta-analytic review testing the stress generation model. *Psychological Bulletin, 149,* 330–369.

Santee, A. C., Rnic, K., Chang, K. K., Chen, R. X., Hoffmeister, J., Liu, H., LeMoult, J., Dozois, D. J. A., & Starr, L. R. (2023). Risk and protective factors for stress generation: A meta-analytic review. *Clinical Psychology Review, 103,* 1–34.

Snyder, D. K., & Whisman, M. A. (Eds.). (2003). *Treating difficult couples: Helping clients with coexisting mental and relationship disorders.* Guilford Press.

Whisman, M. A., & Baucom, D. H. (2012). Intimate relationships and psychopathology. *Clinical Child and Family Psychology Review, 15*(1), 4–13.

Whisman, M. A., Sbarra, D. A., & Beach, S. R. H. (2021). Intimate relationships and depression: Searching for causation in the sea of association. *Annual Review of Clinical Psychology, 17,* 233–258.

Chapter 12. The Power of Negative Thinking

Blais, R. K., & Renshaw, K. D. (2014). Self-stigma fully mediates the association of anticipated enacted stigma and help-seeking intentions in National Guard service members. *Military Psychology, 26*(2), 114–119.

Epstein, N. B., & Falconier, M. K. (2024). *Treatment plans and interventions in couple therapy: A cognitive-behavioral approach.* Guilford Press.

Greenberger, D., & Padesky, C. A. (2016). *Mind over mood: Change how you feel by changing the way you think* (2nd ed.). Guilford Press.

LaBuda, J. E., & Gere, J. (2023). A meta-analytic review of accuracy and bias in romantic partner perceptions. *Psychological Bulletin, 149*(9–10), 580–610.

Lebow, J. L., & Snyder, D. K. (Eds.). (2023). *Clinical handbook of couple therapy* (6th ed.). Guilford Press.

Nichols, M. P., & Straus, M. B. (2021). *The lost art of listening: How learning to listen can improve relationships* (3rd. ed., p. 61). Guilford Press.

Simons, D. J., & Chabris, C. F. (1999). Gorillas in our midst: Sustained inattentional blindness for dynamic events. *Perception, 28*(9), 1059–1074.

Wilde, J., & Dozois, D. J. A. (2019). A dyadic partner-schema model of relationship distress and depression: Conceptual integration of interpersonal theory and cognitive-behavioral models. *Clinical Psychology Review, 70,* 13–25.

Wilde, J., Gillies, J., & Dozois, D. J. A. (2021). Cognitive and interpersonal contributors to relationship distress and depression: A review of the dyadic partner-schema model. In V. R. Preedy, C. Martin, L. A. Hunter, V. Patel, & R. Rajendram (Eds.), *The neuroscience of depression: Cell biology, neurology, behaviour and diet* (pp. 373–380). Elsevier.

Chapter 13. Communication and Problem Solving

Aron, A., Melinat, E., Aron, E. N., Vallone, R. D., & Bator, R. J. (1997). The experimental generation of interpersonal closeness: A procedure and some preliminary findings. *Personality and Social Psychology Bulletin, 23*(4), 363–377.

Baucom, D. H., Epstein, N. B., Fischer, M. S., Kirby, J. S., & LaTaillade, J. J. (2023). Cognitive-behavioral couple therapy. In J. L. Lebow & D. K. Snyder, D. K. (Eds.). *Clinical handbook of couple therapy* (6th ed., pp. 53–78). Guilford Press.

Baucom, D. H., Fischer, M. S., Corrie, S., Worrell, M., & Boeding, S. E. (2019). *Treating relationship distress and psychopathology in couples: A cognitive-behavioural approach.* Routledge.

Catron, M. L. (2015, January 9). To fall in love with anyone, do this. *New York Times.*

Christensen, A., Wheeler, J. G., Doss, B. D., & Jacobson, N. S. (2021). Couple distress. In D. H. Barlow (Ed.), *Clinical handbook of psychological disorders: A step-by-step treatment manual* (6th ed., pp. 742–771). Guilford Press.

Nezu, A. M., Nezu, C. M., Damico, J. L., & Gerber, H. R. (2023). Ineffective social problem solving. In D. J. A. Dozois & K. S. Dobson (Eds.), *Treatment of psychosocial risk factors in depression* (pp. 333–358). American Psychological Association.

Nezu, A. M., Nezu, C. M., & Hays, A. M. (2019). Emotion-centered problem-solving therapy. In K. S. Dobson & D. J. A. Dozois (Eds.), *Handbook of cognitive-behavioral therapies* (4th ed., pp. 171–190). Guilford Press.

Palermo, T. M., Law, E. F, Essner, B., Jessen-Fiddick. T., & Eccleston, C. (2014). Adaptation of problem-solving skills training (PSST) for parent caregivers of youth with chronic pain. *Clinical Practice in Pediatric Psychology, 2*(3), 212–223.

Chapter 14. Acceptance Strategies

Christensen, A., Wheeler, J. G., Doss, B. D., & Jacobson, N. S. (2021). Couple distress. In D. H. Barlow (Ed.), *Clinical handbook of psychological disorders: A step-by-step treatment manual* (6th ed., pp. 742–771). Guilford Press.

Epstein, N. B., & Falconier, M. K. (2024). *Treatment plans and interventions in couple therapy: A cognitive-behavioral approach.* Guilford Press.

Hayes, S. C., Strosahl, K. D., & Wilson, K. G. (2012). *Acceptance and commitment therapy: The process and practice of mindful change* (2nd ed.). Guilford Press.

Lawrence, E., Cohn, A. S., & Allen, S. H. (2023). Acceptance and commitment therapy for couples. In J. L. Lebow & D. K. Snyder (Eds.), *Clinical handbook of couple therapy* (6th ed., pp. 104–124). Guilford Press.

Wegner, D. M., Schneider, D. J., Carter, S. R., & White, T. L. (1987). Paradoxical effects of thought suppression. *Journal of Personality and Social Psychology, 53*(1), 5.

Chapter 15. When Your Partner Improves (or Doesn't Improve)

Aalgaard, R. A., Bolen, R. M., & Nugent, W. R. (2016) A literature review of forgiveness as a beneficial intervention to increase relationship satisfaction in couples therapy, *Journal of Human Behavior in the Social Environment, 26*(1), 46–55.

Baucom, D. H., Epstein, N. B., Fischer, M. S., Kirby, J. S., & LaTaillade, J. J. (2023). Cognitive-behavioral couple therapy. In J. L. Lebow & D. K. Snyder (Eds.), *Clinical handbook of couple therapy* (6th ed., pp. 53–78). Guilford Press.

Baucom, D. H., Fischer, M. S., Corrie, S., Worrell, M., & Boeding, S. E. (2019). *Treating relationship distress and psychopathology in couples: A cognitive-behavioural approach.* Routledge.

Beach, S. R. H., Whisman, M. A., & Bodenmann, G. (2014). Couple, parenting, and interpersonal therapies for depression in adults: Toward common clinical guidelines within a stress-generation framework. In I. H. Gotlib & C. L. Hammen (Eds.), *Handbook of depression* (3rd ed., pp. 552–570). Guilford Press.

Beck, A. T., Rush, A. J., Shaw, B. F., Emery, G., DeRubeis, R. J., & Hollon, S. D. (2024). *Cognitive therapy of depression* (2nd ed.). Guilford Press.

Braithwaite, S. R., Selby, E. A., & Fincham, F. D. (2011). Forgiveness and relationship satisfaction: Mediating mechanisms. *Journal of Family Psychology, 25*(4), 551–559.

Christensen, A., Dimidjian, S., Martell, C. R., & Doss, B. D. (2023). Integrative behavioral couple therapy. In J. L. Lebow & D. K. Snyder (Eds.), *Clinical handbook of couple therapy* (6th ed., pp. 79–103). Guilford Press.

Dozois, D. J. A., & Mental Health Research Canada (2021). Anxiety and depression in Canada during the COVID-19 pandemic: A national survey. *Canadian Psychology, 62,* 136–142.

Epstein, N. B., & Falconier, M. K. (2022). *Treatment plans and interventions in couple therapy: A cognitive-behavioral approach.* Guilford Press.

Flett, G. L. (2018). *The psychology of mattering: Understanding the human need to be significant.* Academic Press.

Johnson, S. M., Wiebe, S. A., & Allan, R. (2023). Emotionally focused couple therapy. In J. L. Lebow & D. K. Snyder (Eds.), *Clinical handbook of couple therapy* (6th ed., pp. 127–150). Guilford Press.

Lam, R. W., Kennedy, S. H., Adams, C., Bahji, A., Beaulieu, S., Bhat, V., Blier, P., Blumberger, D. M., Brietzke, E., Chakrabarty, T., Do, A., Frey, B. N., Giacobbe, P., Gratzer, D., Grigoriadis, S., Habert, J., Ishrat Husain, M., Ismail, Z., McGirr, A., McIntyre, R. S., Michalak, E. E., Müller, D. J., Parikh, S. V., Quilty, L. C., Ravindran, A. V., Ravindran, N., Renaud, J., Rosenblat, J. D., Samaan, Z., Saraf, G., Schade, K., Schaffer, A., Sinyor, M., Soares, C. N., Swainson, J., Taylor, V. H., Tourjman, S. V., Uher, R., van Ameringen M., Vazquez, G., Vigod, S., Voineskos, D., Yatham, L. N., Milev, R. V. (2024). Canadian network for mood and anxiety treatments (CANMAT) 2023 update on clinical guidelines for management of major depressive disorder in adults. *Canadian Journal of Psychiatry, 69*(9), 641–687.

Meneses, C. W., & Greenberg, L. S. (2019). Emotion-focused therapy. In C. W. Meneses & L. S. Greenberg (Eds.), *Forgiveness and letting go in emotion-focused therapy* (pp. 31–50). American Psychological Association.

Mróz, J., & Kaleta, K. (2023). Forgive, let go, and stay well! The relationship between forgiveness and physical and mental health in women and men: The mediating role of self-consciousness. *International Journal of Environmental Research and Public Health, 20*(13), 6229.

Rain, S., & Dozois, D. J. A. (2025). Is precision treatment possible for depression? *Canadian Psychology.* Advance online publication. *https://doi.org/10.1037/cap0000452*

Whisman, M. A., Beach, S. R. H., & Davila, J. (2023). Couple therapy for depression or anxiety. In J. L. Lebow & D. K. Snyder (Eds.), *Clinical handbook of couple therapy* (6th ed., pp. 576–594). Guilford Press.

Whisman, M. A., Johnson, D. P., Be, D., & Li, A. (2012). Couple-based interventions for depression. *Couple and Family Psychology: Research and Practice, 1*(3), 185–198.

World Health Organization. (2024). *COVID-19 dashboard. https://data.who.int/dashboards/covid19/deaths*

Index

Note. *f* following a page number indicates a figure.

About the Author

David J. A. Dozois, PhD, is an internationally known depression researcher and cognitive-behavioral therapist. He is Professor of Psychology at the University of Western Ontario, is a Fellow and two-time president of the Canadian Psychological Association, and has held leadership roles in many other national and international organizations. Dr. Dozois has authored over 300 scientific publications and presents his work widely. He also maintains a small private practice.